UNLEASH YOUR FULL POTENTIAL

by

Matt Espeut

Unleash Your Full Potential

By

Matt Espeut

Visit our website at **www.StillwaterPress.com** for more information.

First Stillwater River Publications Edition

ISBN-10: 1-946-30010-1
ISBN-13: 978-1-946300-10-2

Library of Congress Control Number: 2017934442

1 2 3 4 5 6 7 8 9 10
Written by Matt Espeut
Cover Design by Andy Hunter
Cover Photography by Jessica Pohl

Published by Stillwater River Publications, Glocester, RI, USA.

The views and opinions expressed in this book are solely those of the author and do not necessarily reflect the views and opinions of the publisher.

DEDICATION

Mom and Dad, for all their love and encouragement over the years, and for providing me with a no quit attitude and a strong work ethic.

Bob Chesney, for telling me I was skinny and needed to start lifting with him. Now I am concerned with Bob's health, and want to help him get back in shape again.

Nancy Thomas, for all her introductions, and helping me build my local platform and network of people.

The owners of Gold's Gym, where I started my career as a trainer.

Dino Campopiano, the head coach of the Shea High School football team, for giving me a coaching opportunity.

Artie Artwell, my boxing and fitness coach for the last 20 years.

My top four mentors, who are:

> Paul Chek for my holistic health back ground.

> Martin Rooney for his high energy and motivation to be a great coach.

> Todd Durkin for his inspiration to be better at everything in life.

> Bedros Keuilian for all his motivation and business coaching.

And to all my past and present clientele who trusted me to help them improve their physical well-being, as well as referring me to others for the same. I couldn't have done it without you.

TABLE OF CONTENTS

SECTION TWO: BODY & FITNESS

FOREWORD

Matt had a dream. His dream wasn't to own a gym or become successful in business. It was to restore people to good health.

For over 25 years, clients from ages fourteen to eighty-six have benefitted from life changes under Matt's direction. These changes go way beyond the technical part of exercise. Matt works with the whole person, and his advice and counsel include nutrition and a healthy mindset. Overall health, strength, and functional conditioning have always been his focus, and today, as a successful owner of a Fit Body Boot Camp franchise in Rhode Island, his dream has allowed other people to make their dreams come true, too.

What will you read in this book? You will read advice that is straight from the hip — he tells it as it is — recognizing that life pulls on us, this way and that, but that you cannot allow excuses to stand in the way of your goals.

Matt's dedication to educating people starts with his nephew and his Boy Scout troop, and extends to Arthur, an octogenarian client who comes to work with him in street shoes and khakis. Never hesitating to help others, Matt shares his advice with people in a local online blog, on the radio, by speaking, writing for publications, and each day in his very active social media presence. Going to where the people are, rather than waiting for them to come to him, makes him unique in this world where so many are only concerned with making a buck as their ultimate goal, not making people happy and healthy — which is Matt's ultimate goal.

On a personal basis, Matt walks the walk and talks the talk, that's for sure. His own fitness as a late-40s man stands as an example to those he instructs. The occasional modeling gig further demonstrates all life can be when you have your health and proper mindset.

When you hear someone say, "hey, they're the real deal," you might wonder what that means. As you read this book, think about that phrase, because that is what you are getting — not a weight loss gimmick or a funky plan of some sort to give you temporary success or a looking-good fix. What you will get is a lifetime plan — one that will give you the knowledge and the motivation to not only look good, but to stay healthy. Who are you doing that for? Well, first, for yourself, Matt would say. But he'd also say, do this for those who love you — and those you are responsible for — your family, parents, and children. They deserve to have you around a very long time. In doing so, you will be a role model for them, too. And that's how we change the world.

Nancy Thomas
President
Tapestry Communications

INTRODUCTION

"Who the hell is Matt Espeut? ," somebody replied to a friend's Facebook post after the friend told someone else to "ask Matt Espeut" when inquiring about fitness. So in case you don't know who I am, and what I'm about, and why I do what I do, read on…

I'm the guy who has helped hundreds of people lose thousands of pounds. That's right — thousands. I have been a personal trainer for over 25 years, and I have helped hundreds of people get fit and lose unwanted body fat. I have worked with hundred-pound losers, and many others have lost high double digits. Now that I have opened Providence Fit Body Boot Camp, I can help even more. Just in the last year alone, I have taken on over a hundred new clients and have been helping them achieve amazing results, so that total is rising rapidly. I keep track!

I'm the guy on a mission to help thousands more achieve amazing fitness and fat loss results. Before I had my own gym, I was limited to what I could do training people one on one. When I worked for another gym, my hands were tied with the number of people I could reach on a daily basis, but now that I have my own place, I'm on the rise, and currently see as many as 150 people a day. I run nine sessions daily, and I am capable of handling 30 at a time, helping more people achieve their goals, and still have time for individual attention and nutrition plans.

I deliver a no-nonsense approach to health and fitness. The first step is to cure a negative mindset, and help you believe that you can accomplish your goals regardless of your situation. I don't accept excuses, and I always have a counter punch ready for you when you fabricate one for yourself. I make it simple for you to achieve, but not easy. I tell you straight up that this requires hard work and discipline and a positive mindset, and there is no simple fix or magic bullet. All you need to do is show up three to five times per week, follow a simple nutrition plan, drink lots of water, get adequate rest, and you are on your way. When you show up to a workout, you will work hard, but you'll do it safely, efficiently, and have some fun while doing it.

So, I like to think of myself as that guy who owns Providence's best results-driven gym. There are other programs cheaper, even bargain basement specials at $10 a month, but all you are paying for is access to a bunch of sophisticated equipment. I think of it like a Rent-A-Center for gym equipment. You get time in the gym, but not much personal attention or knowledge provided on what to do with all that. Not here. As a matter of fact, you will not see a single piece of equipment in my facility that requires electricity. We base our workouts on functional strength and metabolic conditioning, using a variety of bodyweight movements, with simple resistance equipment such as battle ropes, medicine balls, dumbbells, free weight barbells, Plyo boxes, sand bags, and resistance tubing. The stuff that gets you real results. No treadmills, elliptical trainers, and recumbent bikes. We also structure and coach our workouts so you are actually working out the whole time you are here. Not watching television, or checking your phone.

I care

I care, and I do everything I can to get you the results you sign up for. There are a lot of gym owners out there, or chain facilities, who care until you make the first payment. And you might not ever seem them working out themselves. They don't walk the walk, or talk the talk — but I do. I stay with you through your journey until you achieve success. I will follow up with your nutrition plan, and send constant emails to you so you stay focused. Yes, I am a pain in your derriere, but that's what you signed up for... results.

I am certified and constantly go to continuing training. I'm one of a large group of pros from all around the country who share information with each other about techniques and programs that work — that keep you motivated and constantly moving closer to your goals. So when you finally decide that you are tired of messing around with fitness routines that don't work, or you are tired of wasting valuable time and hard-earned money on programs that get you nowhere, who are you gonna call? After you work with me awhile, maybe you can leave a testimonial on my Facebook page so that guy who asked that question will know exactly who I am.

UNLEASH YOUR
FULL POTENTIAL

SECTION ONE

MIND
& SPIRIT

1

THREE THINGS
TO STOP SAYING —
TODAY!

I am always writing about what things you can do to improve your current health and fitness situation, but today I have come up with a few things you should *stop* doing to improve your health and fitness, or in fact, to improve anything in your life.

Stop saying "I don't have the time."

We all have 24 hours in a day and 168 hours in a week, so it's just a matter of organizing your time and prioritizing the things that are important to get done. Did you understand that last line? The "important" things are not the things you "feel" like doing, but are the things you need to be doing. They should be at the top of your daily list. When you organize your day, you will find that the time to do the things you need to do will be there. If your excuse for not working out is time, then your health and wellness are not priorities in your life. You are basically saying, "I am not worth investing 3 out of 168 hours this week to take care of myself." If you watch any television, spend hours on social media, take long lunches, or gossip with friends on the phone, well then, you do have the time — you just choose to waste it with things that aren't "important." So

1

stop using the term, "I didn't have time," and instead replace it with the line, "I didn't get it done because it wasn't a priority."

Stop saying "I am trying."

"I am trying," is a soft way of saying "I am NOT doing it." When someone says, "I am trying to eat better," they are really saying, "I have no will power and discipline, I am weak, and I do not feel like giving 100 percent to a good nutrition plan." There is no "trying" to eat healthy; you either do it or you don't. There isn't anybody knocking carrots out of your hand and forcing cupcakes down your throat, or following you to the supermarket and making you buy junk food. This is not a hard concept. You have to eat, and it's all your decision to eat right or not. If you truly try to do something, you will be "doing it" and not "trying to do it." If you were trying to win a gold medal in the Olympics, and you kept falling fractions of a second short, you have the right to say, "I keep trying for gold, but keep earning silver." But if you fall short of eating healthy and getting to the gym, you aren't trying hard enough.

Stop saying "It's not my fault."

Sigmund Freud once said, "Most people don't want freedom, because freedom comes with responsibility."

Be responsible for your own actions, and don't blame others for what you are doing or going through, because when you deny responsibility, you are surrendering control over your own life. Take control of your life and accept responsibility for your own actions. You are in full control of how you choose to deal with the current state of your life. Blaming your spouse, parents, or co-workers is just another way to transfer falling short of your goals onto others. Stop saying "but it's not my fault," because it is. If you want to change, then get healthy, and you'll succeed at anything. It's up to you. The only person who can make it happen is you!

If you remove these terms from your vocabulary, success in whatever you set out to do will become more likely. I have a rule that I follow, and it is to never complain about time or anything time related. I try to structure my day with a priority list, and I find that I get my important tasks done 99 percent of the time. If I didn't get something done, I say "That wasn't a priority, and I used my time for something else," not "I didn't have the time," because that would be a lie. When someone suddenly gets sick, or has an accident, you miraculously find the time to help them. You would never say, "I don't have time to drive you to the emergency room or visit you in the hospital." You make it a priority, and the time is used taking care of that priority.

If things in life, like fitness and success were easy, everyone would be doing them. It's much easier to use these excuses for failing, and that's why obesity, disease, and poverty are at an all-time high. It's all about mindset, discipline, and execution. Program yourself to be a doer and an action taker, and stop hiding behind excuses. Think to yourself that if others can do it, then so can you. We are all in the same boat with pretty much the same opportunities, all with the same amount of time in the day. What separates us are the decisions we make and how we choose to spend our time.

How will you spend your time today?

2

5... 4... 3... 2... 1... Go!

Give yourself a countdown. Don't just jump straight in on day one of your new nutrition and exercise program. Remember, your biggest predictor of success will be if your mindset is where it needs to be. So, think about what you are doing. And think about all the reasons you are doing it. Visualize your goal. Imagine long and hard what that will be like to achieve it. Sure, it's OK to think of vanity first — your clothes will fit better, you will look better — but also think about your body and how you'll feel better, maybe you'll even be able to get off some of your high blood pressure or pre-diabetes meds. Think about the message you will be sending your family and your children. Let that stew around in your thoughts for five days before you start.

For many of us, setting arbitrary goals and start dates do help us prepare for success. As with other lifestyle changes such as stopping smoking, for example, 90 percent of your success comes from your decision process — have you truly decided to "do this" — and are you fully committed to it? That starts today. Here are some tips to help you do the five-day countdown to being fit for life.

Day Five — Today

Start the psychological wheels turning about your fitness goals. What do you want to accomplish? Look better? Feel better? Be healthier? Live longer? Get stronger to avoid injury at work? Spend some time thinking about the "why." And it's OK to do it for someone else — your children, your spouse, your family, or even your job. More than thinking, you should visualize what life will be like for you when you are well on your way to your goal. What will your day look like? How will it change? What will you do that you can't do now? Use all your senses to wrap yourself around that feeling. If you meditate, use visualizations. Talk out loud about your goals to those who will be part of helping you get there but not undermining your success. As with many good and enjoyable things, it all starts in your mind. Make this a powerful tool to success.

Day Four

Today is research day. Read good sources of information. Spend some time on the internet. Don't go to those beat-down sites, as I call them, because most of those quick and easy plans won't work for you; they might in the beginning, but not long term. And isn't that what you are striving for? If you succeed now, you will be in "maintenance mode" not "life changing mode" all the time. Talk to your friends who you admire for their fitness levels and good eating habits. What do they do? What will you enjoy doing? Remember — a gym membership is not an answer, it's just a tool like any other tool you use. But if you truly hate your workout choice, you won't stick with it. So, gather the info, print articles, cut out magazine stories, and sit back with a cup of green tea and think about your options.

Day Three

Going cold turkey is tough. For anyone. And, as I've said over and over again, you can't work out a bad diet. Take a look at what you eat. Start a journal to document and really capture all that you eat, not only food, but drink and snacks. You'll want to note what *type* of food you are eating, too. Are there GMOs (Genetically Modified Organisms) in your diet? Get rid of 'em. Read the labels. Clean your cabinets of junk. Ban the soda, the power drinks, and especially the caffeine boosting drinks. Get a water filter. Or buy bottled water.

Americans eat far too much — and usually the wrong things. It's OK to pile up your plate, but it should be with veggies, some fruit, and good sources of protein, not mounds of carbs, or gravies, or fatty foods. Browse a supermarket with healthy selections. Buy a cookbook. If you commit to eating sensibly, you shouldn't have to spend a fortune to do this. Think about bringing healthy lunches to work, quick things you can eat for breakfast, good-for-you snacks and your main meals. Buy a crockpot so you can come home and find a healthy dinner, ready and waiting for you. You will now be on your way to eating healthy, good, real food — your power source to success.

Day Two

Do some shopping. Do you have functional sneakers for your workout? There are different designs for walking, running, etc. If going outdoors will be part of your routine, and of course if it's winter, you'll want to get natural fiber (cotton, wool) hat, scarf, and gloves. Cover your mouth and nose with a scarf when it's bitterly cold. Buy some lightweight clothes to layer on — there are some expensive items out there that will wick the sweat away from your body — but remember, you don't *need* these, they are an extra tool. Do you have comfortable sweatpants or shorts for the gym? Will you be showering there? You'll want to make up a gym bag of items that you can take back and forth, like soap and shampoo. If mobile apps and pedometers will help you keep your commitment to fitness, go right ahead and get them. Now you have everything you need. Relax, get ready, then go to sleep in a happy way because you know what tomorrow will bring — the beginning of a whole new YOU.

Day One

It's here. You have everything you need. You have your plan, your things, and your tools. Write it all down today. Spell out your goals in writing. If you need help from a personal trainer, or someone to take you grocery shopping, remember — good personal trainers will do more than work you out in a gym. So, let's review. You have your stuff — clothes, equipment, tools. You have your food, some recipes and cookbooks. You've tossed the junk food and junk drinks out of your house. You have a plan and you know what type of exercise you will start with, even if it's just walking on the first day.

Remember to keep variety in your workout to keep your interest and to mix up your muscles for maximum benefit. Now — as with everything — your success starts at the beginning. *Your commitment.* If you truly have embraced being more fit, healthier and happier this year — and beyond — it starts with a solid decision to do so. You may have to revisit this along the way and recommit, if you slip. But don't be hard on yourself, just get right back up and continue on. Good Luck — my wish for you is to be FIT FOR LIFE — and it starts today — 5, 4, 3, 2, 1 — GO!

3

BE A PRO

Why be mediocre? Why be average? Rise and conquer! Be a professional. Do your best at everything, and success will follow. I was out sledding with my nephew last weekend, and we were at a place that attracts a lot of people — different ages, sizes, races, and religions. And I started to notice how some people were dressed for the frigid cold, wet weather we were experiencing. Some kids were wearing nothing but a pair of pajama bottoms, sneakers, and a hooded sweatshirt. As for us, we both had snow pants, weather appropriate boots, and were dressed in layers. As the day went on, I noticed how uncomfortable, cranky, and cold the others were, but not us. We were having a blast! I told a friend about the situation, and she replied, "You guys had more fun because you were dressed like professionals." It was then I started thinking: whatever it is you do, you will do it better and enjoy it more if you take the time to prepare and be a professional about it. This holds true with everything from sledding, to work, to exercise, to a day at the beach — and taking care of your health.

A pro at work

Let's use work as a first example: When you express passion, enthusiasm, and take the time to prepare, you will like your job better, perform it more efficiently, and ultimately make more money than someone who is careless, unmotivated, and unprepared to tackle the tasks at hand. Unless you show up at work as a professional, you will be considered just another worker, and probably be over-looked for advancement, thus making your profession laborious, boring, and unsatisfying. You won't have all that much pride in what you do, and will end up hating your job, which will make life a miserable existence. I don't care what you do, whether you work at a drive thru or are the CEO of a corporation, when you approach things and act like a pro, good things will come your way.

A pro at fun

Another good example would be a day at the beach. You know that if you take the time to pack a lunch, sunscreen, a chair, books, and a clean change of clothes, you are guaranteed to enjoy your day more than someone who doesn't plan, but just grabs a towel to sit on — he'll have a day of sitting in sand, getting a painful sunburn, eating fried clams, hotdogs and chips from the snack bar, then driving home in a wet bathing suit. Sound appealing to you? Not to me. But it does sound like a failure to prepare.

A pro at fitness

So what can we learn to apply to exercising and your health? If you schedule your workouts, eat properly, get plenty of rest and wear the right gear, you will not only enjoy the concept of taking care of yourself, but the results will show much more than someone who wears the wrong gear, never shops for food, always eats on the go, and has no commitment to getting to the gym on a regular basis. These are the fly-by-nighters. They do it half-assed, complain about how hard it is, and never get the outcome they envisioned for themselves. These people fall in the amateur category. They constantly start things and never follow through. They workout but do not eat properly, or they eat a few good meals and then fall off the wagon at night. This happens because of their mindset.

My advice is simple — you will never be good at anything unless you exert some effort, time, and a desire to be better. You can't put things low on your priority list and expect to excel at them. When people join my Fit Body Boot Camp, I allow them unlimited access to my session schedule, give them a solid nutrition plan, weigh and measure them, and hold them accountable. I supply all the tools they need to succeed. The members who have the right mindset put time into preparing their meals, show up regularly, and work hard. They not only get results, but they are actually happy to be there. You can feel it in their posts on my Facebook page. Reading their positive notes and how they feel about their improving bodies by working with me makes my day too. I've also noticed that the more people get into better shape, the nicer workout clothes and sneakers they start wearing. Why? Because the results are addictive. The more you achieve, the better you feel, and it makes you want to look better both inside and out. In other words, they have stepped out of the amateur ranks, and show up looking and acting like — *professionals*!

4

BE OBSESSIVE!
IT'S A GOOD THING.

For years I have been hearing people say "You're too obsessive when it comes to fitness, " or "You're too obsessive when you buy food or are about to eat," or "You need to relax and live a little," or "You're too competitive." I am now OVER 40 years-old, and I am in the best shape of my life. And not only do I feel great, but I have my blood work done every year, and the results are always far above average. Am I really obsessive? Hell yes! Am I going to continue to be obsessive about everything I do that's important to me? MOST DEFINITELY!

Many people think of obsessions as something bad, unhealthy, or problematic. In my opinion, if you aren't obsessive about the things you do, you are only going to do things half-way and will never reach your full potential. That's fine if you want to be average at what you do; but being average isn't in my play book.

If NASA wasn't obsessive, would we have put a man on the moon? If Tom Brady wasn't obsessive, would he go down as one of the greatest quarterbacks of all time? If Barack Obama wasn't driven by obsession, would he have become the first Black president? If Thomas Edison didn't obsess about inventing things, would he have been successful? And if Steve Jobs wasn't obsessive, would Apple be where it is today? NO, NO, NO, and NO! And let me give

11

you a little news flash: if you are not obsessive about the things that are important to you in your life, success will elude you on every level whether it be fitness, finances, or family matters. If you don't have obsession, passion, and drive you will either fail, become mediocre, or be average at best.

Will you accept being average?

We live in a world where people accept being average. But where does this get us? High unemployment, high obesity rate, record levels of poverty, poor education among our population, and people looking for the easy way out. Lack of obsession and drive is what has caused these things, not bad luck, foul weather, or the government. It's the lack of drive, discipline and desire to better oneself, or lack of obsession, that causes us to be lazy and not accomplish things. Still think being obsessive is a bad thing? I think it's necessary to succeed.

My newest obsession is to build my new business to its highest level possible. I want to reach the point where I dominate the fitness industry in our state. I want to have so many fitness and fat loss success stories that when you hear fitness, health, get in shape, great workout programs, and results mentioned — Matt Espeut and Providence Fit Body Boot Camp immediately come to mind. And I am on my way. I listen and read self-help, personal growth, and success books whenever I can. I fly coast to coast to attend seminars and conferences hosted by the best in the business so I can be with like-minded people and learn from them. I work day and night to bring my clients the best services and programs I can, and to generate new clients to help. I am thinking every hour I am awake on how to improve and grow, and I don't plan on stopping until my mission is done. And I believe without obsession, it wouldn't be happening!

Let's obsess together

So there you have it people. Take it for what it is. Want to get in shape? Then be obsessive about it. You won't get fit and healthy exercising one day a week, and eating healthy — sometimes. You won't get promoted, by going to work and working hard — once in a while. You won't become a good golfer if you only play — a few times a season. And you won't be a good parent if you only pay attention to your kids — sometimes.

So, stop shedding a negative image on people that have a vision, work hard, and focus on succeeding. Instead, get your butt off the sofa, come on down to my gym, and let's obsess together about making you fit and healthy.

5

BRING YOUR "A" GAME

Why reward someone for doing something wrong? Are my expectations too high, or has society lowered their standards too much? I was leaving a coffee shop the other day when a very overweight individual lumbered by in a futile attempt to run at a fitness level. Someone gave him a fist pump and said, "Good for you!" I couldn't help asking, "what's so good?" The reply was, "well, at least he's trying." So, I went on and explained that he was actually doing more harm than good. Granted, I received a confused look and was asked what I meant. So, I went on to explain that he was exercising with very bad form and technique — he had a forward head tilt, bad posture, incorrect contact with the ground and bad hand position. I went on further to say that in this one instance, he would have been better off doing nothing rather than most likely causing eventual harm or injury to his body.

To me, trying isn't going to get you where you want to be unless you have a plan and execute it properly. Just randomly trying to do something you know nothing about will net zero results and just waste your time. This is true for most things in life where you don't possess the expertise to accomplish your task or goal. It's like trying to climb a mountain without the necessary equipment, knowledge, or experience. At best, you will only waste your time or be embarrassed while failing. At worst, you will get hurt.

I don't give credit for trying in this instance, but if you were properly prepared, and then failed, I would give you credit for trying. The definition of trying is to "make an attempt or effort to do something (strive) or to do one's best." When you just randomly go through the motions with half an effort, that doesn't constitute trying. No credit should be given until you legitimately give something a "try." I have a brother with self-induced diabetes, and anytime we eat at family dinners, I get on him for eating dessert and high sugar items. He always lashes back at me to leave him alone, "I am trying to eat better." I always come back with, "If you want credit for trying, then really try. Don't eat sweets."

Trying? Or... Doing!

I believe that if you really give your best with a 100 percent effort, then you won't be saying, "I'm trying"; instead you'll be saying, "I'm doing!" I had a great experience at a restaurant last weekend, and when I left, I marveled at how great the service was, and how the waitress was well-tuned into food and gluten, and how well the dishes were prepared. She was on the ball from start to finish, and when the meal came out, the owner personally brought it to my table and asked if everything was to my liking. The food was great quality (grass fed beef), came out in a timely manner, and was prepared perfectly. After I left, I was talking to some friends, and in a tone of voice that sounded nothing short of "surprising," I told them how great the experience was. I found myself stepping back to wonder, why it's so shocking when we receive great quality? Isn't that how it is always supposed to be? All the time? Most of the time? You see, that goes back to my only praising when things are 100 percent on point. I don't give credit for attempts, or partial completion. The same goes for fitness. You won't get credit for just showing up, but neither will you won't get results going at it half way, or just going through the motions. So, let's step it up people, and put your best effort forward. Bring out your "A" game every day.

6

CHANGE. EMBRACE IT.

L ast week I talked about insanity, and wasting time, by doing the same thing over and over without getting favorable results. I gave an example of how to avoid this by hiring a coach and letting the expert lead you through unfamiliar territory. This is a good way to efficiently reach your goals, but there is one big obstacle we need to overcome before this can work and be effective, and that obstacle is YOU. Hiring the best coach in the world will not get you results unless you are coachable and willing to change. If you are unable or unwilling to do this, save your money and stop wasting your time.

I admit, I do have an old-school mentality, and I do prefer a time when things were less complicated, especially in the fast-moving world of technology. But I realized that if I didn't change I would be left behind and out of touch with the business world. The words "evolve or die" carry great importance to me, and that saying has helped open my eyes and realize that all change isn't bad. I explained this to my mother when she would get upset that my nephew's teachers didn't "call" every parent when something happened or changed at school. I explained that sending one email was far more efficient than making 500 phone calls. She got it, and now has an iPhone and texts people all the time!

You need to be willing and able to be coached if you want change to happen. I have trained numerous people who have difficulty making changes to their lifestyle and habits, and that gives me great difficulty getting them the results they want. I usually start a relationship with a client by saying that I am only with them 2-3 hours a week, and what they do with the other 165 is just as, if not, more critical than our time together in the gym. I let them know that unless they change their eating, sleeping and exercise habits, I can't do much more than give them a good workout and good advice. "Help me help you," I tell them. You supply the discipline, I will supply the knowledge, and together we can make it happen. If they are willing, it happens; if not, it doesn't. Most of the time it is easier and the results come faster with someone new to exercising because they are a blank slate and I do not need to change bad exercise habits and movement patterns. I have worked with people coming from other trainers and coaches and hear, "But my other trainer did this, or my high school coach said that." If it makes sense I will listen, but most of the time it doesn't, and I give an obnoxious reply like "Obviously, that didn't work, so let's do it my way."

Even as a professional, change is necessary if you want to be the best at what you do. Mike Boyle is a coach and presenter from Boston who tells it like it is and bluntly says, "If you know an exercise isn't great, or even worse, harmful, and you keep doing it because everyone uses it or it is something you always do, you are a moron." He humbly admits that he had clients doing exercises that he discovered were wrong or not beneficial and quit doing them. His philosophy is that a good coach will change for the benefit of his clients or players, and not let his ego dictate his actions. This is from an expert who trains trainers and coaches. Ten years ago, I was putting my clients on leg press/extension, and numerous other weight machines, because they were new, smooth, shiny and cool looking, and everyone was using them. Did they isolate and make your muscles bigger? Yes. Did they cause imbalances, joint pain, and feed postural dysfunction? Yes! So guess what? I haven't put a client on a weight machine in over 10 years. Your muscles will respond just as well, if not better, doing free standing squats, or moving dumbbells, and free weights. The human body should still move and function the way it did hundreds of years ago.

So when you seek out a professional coach to help you with whatever it is you want to accomplish, remember: you sought help because your way wasn't working. Make life a lot easier for yourself and your coach and be ready not only to MAKE changes, but to embrace them.

7

CINDERELLA WAS SKINNY-FAT

As Disney parades yet another princess movie before our children, what message are young boys and girls getting? Ladies, if you want to be beautiful — *no, if you want to be a PRINCESS* — then be slim. Be slimmer than slim — be skinny. And even if you are super thin, wear a corset and suck it in to an unrealistic waist to body ratio. Boys, do you want to marry the princess? All you have to do is watch an awards program like the Oscars or Emmys and you'll see it — the celebrities are super thin and talking all about how they can't wait to eat after the show. Those who have anything on under their skin-tight gowns will admit to wearing three layers of Spanx. They've been dieting to fit into the extraordinarily tight gowns — and it shows. Women who have had babies literally weeks before are now magically restored to princess quality.

The actress Lily James (who plays Cinderella in the newest movie,) admitted to having to stay on a liquid diet to fit into the corset under her costumes, going on to say, "If I ate food, it didn't really digest properly, and I'd be burping all afternoon... it was just really sort of unpleasant. I'd have soup so that I could still eat but it wouldn't get stuck," she said. "The corset pulled me (within an) inch of my life."

Being overweight is unhealthy, but so is being unnaturally thin. You are literally skinny-fat (as much as I don't like the term "fat").

If you are a woman, sized 4 and your arms and legs jiggle because your skin is hanging off the bone, this can be you. Your BMI can be very much like that of an overweight person, too. You can also have high cholesterol, be pre-diabetic or what I see most often, have mysterious food allergies and sensitivities. Here's how you probably got that way:

* You do too much cardio

* You do not get enough rest

* You do not do strength training

* You starve yourself / cut calories

* You are regularly dehydrated

Want to be a beautiful, healthy woman?

* Lay off cardio & let your body heal. Stop wasting valuable nutrients your body needs to gain muscle.

* Strength training and building muscle will make you tone and fit and aesthetically more appealing.

* Eat the proper nutrients. You cannot build muscle without the proper raw materials.

* Rest. Your body cannot utilize nutrients and repair damaged cells without sleep.

* Drink quality water and hydrate your body.

Now carry that message to the children in your family. It will help to raise empowered young women who value health as the measure of their beauty, first and foremost. And young men will value this too — opting for strength and health over insecure, unhealthy, look-obsessed princesses.

8

DES·TI·NY

DESTINY: destinē/noun
1. the events that will necessarily happen to a particular person or thing in the future; "she was unable to control her own destiny"
2. the hidden power believed to control what will happen in the future; fate; "he believes in destiny"

This is the definition of DESTINY. The first definition states the truth, but I tend to disagree with the second one on many levels.

Are there things in life we can't control?

Absolutely. There are many chronic illnesses and diseases that are beyond our control, and many times there is nothing we could have done to change an outcome, even if we knew it was going to happen. But when it comes to our health and wellness, I believe we can control 90 percent of all that ails us, and WE, not some hidden power, have control over this. Very few human beings have sickness and ill health as part of their destiny. If we take some time and apply some effort, we should be able to live a healthy vital life.

I am writing this while sitting bedside with a family member in the hospital, and I am surrounded by sickness and death. The person I am visiting is looking at a 50/50 chance of survival due to an episode that could have definitely been avoided. This is someone who knew he was sick, knew what to do to get better (because I always nag him), yet never made the effort or took the time to take care of himself, not realizing the consequences that go along with an unhealthy lifestyle. The scary part is that this isn't uncommon. I see it and hear about it every day, and I can't understand why.

We see it everywhere. People eating poorly, not exercising, and doing abusive things to their body. And look what they have to show for it — obesity, heart disease, arthritis, respiratory problems, medication dependency, poor self-image, low energy... and the list goes on and on and on.

The domino effect

Not only does this effect the individual not taking care of themselves, it creates a domino effect. Families suffer while watching it take place, and they will suffer even more when an untimely death occurs. It is torture when someone you care about is damaging themselves to the point you expect a disastrous outcome to their lives. It also causes a huge increase in the cost of medical care. Hospitals are expensive, and you can purchase many organic foods and gym memberships with the cost of one stint in the hospital.

Do it for those you love

So in conclusion, if your destiny is to be sick, feel lousy, and be unproductive in your life, all while upsetting those around you who care about you, then keep eating packaged processed junk, smoking cigarettes, drinking alcohol and not exercising. Many of the people doing this don't realize the repercussions, so if this describes you, (my younger brother) please take note and make some changes in your life. Many of you have families and children, so even if you don't care about yourself, consider those around you. We care and want what's best for you. If you are serious about making a change for the better, call me at Providence Fit Body Boot Camp, and I'll help you.

9

BACK TO SCHOOL —
TWO WAYS TO
GET IT RIGHT

P arents rejoice when it's back to school time for the young ones! But, I believe this is a critical time — a moment when natural new patterns are all in motion. You get to watch them get excited about new clothes, sneakers, and being back with their friends. But there are a couple things that kids don't care about that but you should: 1) their nutrition; and, 2) if they play sports, their training. Realistically, most school lunches contain nothing but processed garbage or extremely poor-quality food, and most kids that play sports do not get enough organized training to prepare them for their specific activity. Here are a few tips on how to combat both dilemmas.

First, nutrition

Start with a fundamental question: What will I absolutely not include in their lunch bags? This is an important question. Folks will find their own way, but many of the items advertised for lunch boxes are processed crap masquerading as sustenance. We know that it's unhealthy; we know it's addictive, yet we still see these items marketed to us. It may have "as much calcium as an 8-oz. glass of milk," but Kraft doesn't trumpet the trans fats, artificial dyes and other nasty stuff in the ingredients. Here's what is in that "cheese:"

> *Nonfat Milk, Water, Sugar, Modified Corn Starch,* **Partially Hydrogenated Soybean Oil**, *less than 2% of: Cocoa (Processed with Alkali), Salt, Calcium Carbonate, Sodium Stearoyl Lactylate, Natural and Artificial Flavors,* **Yellow 5, Yellow 6.**

That isn't the nutrition you want your kids gobbling, so you should not be including anything like this on their menu. Once we have the framework down of what we will not feed them, then we discuss what we will include. I ask two questions: Will it make you proud when you've packed it all up that you've done your job of giving them a great lunch and snacks? And here's an important question — will they eat it? I understand the balance between healthy and convenient, flexible and diligent, aware and open. You can pack the world's healthiest lunch, but it does no good if your kids won't eat it. Even if you have to make peanut butter and jelly, purchase the highest quality bread that your child will eat, but without those "no chance" items like high fructose corn syrup, artificial colors, etc. Always get a jelly that's mostly fruit and as natural organic a peanut butter as possible. But even high quality PB & J only takes us so far. To really plan out a menu, before school starts, have a family meeting. Ask your kids what they would like to see in their lunches this year. If you can't get a straight answer, you need to go straight to the grocery store and walk up and down the aisles together. This way you can make informed decisions and it won't feel like you are forcing good healthy food on them. Get them excited about fresh fruits, tasty vegetables like carrots, healthy trail mixes, and quality deli meats, and breads. This will make them happy and you will be satisfied that you are doing a good job as a parent, and that your kids are really eating healthier.

Athletics & Training

Now that we've addressed some nutrition issues, let's talk about athletics. Think on the pro level. What do the pros do in the off-season? They train. Not only for strength and performance, but also for conditioning and injury prevention. Why treat kids differently? When untrained athletes take the field, they are doubling their chance of injury, as well as getting their ego, and self-esteem pummeled, because they can't compete. You don't need to send your kids off to some expensive showcase, or training camp; just a few workout sessions per week will help improve their overall conditioning. Beware if they hit the gym with their friends, usually they will grab a suggested workout exercise idea out of a magazine and attempt it on their own. Not only will they increase their odds of getting injured, they may gain absolutely nothing because of improper technique. The best advice I can give a parent is to hire a trained professional with experience in sports training. When I train my youth athletes, my number one concern is weakness in their core, and my second concern is that they are still growing and developing, so many are extremely awkward. Special attention needs to be paid, because an adolescent should develop their core before loading the body. Movement patterns need to be perfected, before speed work is implemented. Progressions need to be strategically planned so imbalances, dysfunction, and injury do not occur. I am not a parent, but every parent I know wants their child to excel, and will cringe and feel the pain when their kid gets hurt. These issues can be solved by implementing a simple training program, so if you want to have your child be competitive, and injury free, include some good nutrition and training to that back to school schedule. It'll keep everyone happy all year through, and have you feeling that success that you felt on their first day back.

10

WE ARE A
DIVIDED NATION

Half conservative, half liberal. Half for gun-control, half against it. We are divided by different faiths and religions, which dictates many different views on issues such as abortion, contraception and same sex marriage. We also have different views on issues like who gets taxed and who doesn't, and which group is entitled to certain social programs, and which ones aren't. It is common that when a person is on one side of any of these issues, they are usually on the same side across the board. Kind of like a "master lever" of opinions held.

However, there is one issue that has no political or religious team, and that's concern about one's health. There is no discrimination, political party, race, sex or religion that separates the two sides. This division is the healthy and the unhealthy people of this nation. And the numbers aren't even close.

Those who are unfit and in poor health are outnumbering the fit and healthy by a landslide. Rather than approach health in a preventive frame of mind, people would rather get sick, and then react. There are issues and debates that can be seen from both sides, but I can't comprehend the decision to be unhealthy. I am not talking about the misinformed, or people who think they are trying only to be fooled by big marketing of commercial foods and weight loss gimmicks, or the people who are on low salt and low-fat garbage because their doctor told them that their blood pressure or cholesterol was too high. I am talking about the people who deliberately use drive-thru windows as their primary food source. Most often, these are the same people who protest the mayor of New York City for banning big gulp sodas. They do not want the government or anybody else telling them how to live, even if it is in everyone's best interest. These are the people who are making a conscious choice to be ignorant of the evidence — they are literally choosing to be or become unhealthy, going down the road of killing themselves slowly, with no consideration for loved ones, much less concern for healthcare costs for themselves or the country. This puts a burden on everyone in many ways, and I will give you a quick example of how this ignorance and choice impacts all of us.

When you let yourself go, eat processed garbage, and don't exercise, it's not a question of IF you will get sick, but WHEN you will get sick. When you do, you clog up the medical system with what are preventable ailments. Once you get into the system, and get on prescription drugs, you become a prisoner for life. When this happens, hospitals become a revolving door, and we all get hit in the pocketbook because insurance is based on averages.

So the people who care about their health and well-being, and choose healthy lifestyles, get to pay unnecessarily high premiums so insurance and medical companies can recoup the payouts from the other side. I know I can't reach everyone, and it is impossible for everyone to think on the same level, but it is extremely frustrating to watch people do deliberate harm to themselves. I can't seem to get the rationale behind killing yourself slowly. I understand that there are addictions, and the lure of sugar, carbohydrates and fat is real — and that it is hard to adhere to a strict program, and I try to not to chastise anyone in this category; my issue is with those who know — and do not care. They lobby against everything that could help put a strain on fake food manufacturers, prevent dangerous drugs from being on the shelves, or try to clean up the school lunch programs. These people are standing in the way of making changes for the better. They represent the demand for harmful products, and keep these unscrupulous companies rich and powerful.

So if you care about your health, but are stuck in a rut, let's talk. If you just do not care, love feeling lethargic with aches and pains, or are overweight and out of shape, by all means keep killing yourself; but please stop trying to interfere with those efforts that will help those of us who do care. I'm talking about those who want bans on soft drinks, and high taxes on sugar, cigarettes, and alcohol. We want the schools to intervene and remove soda machines, processed nugget-food, and fake cheese from the selections. I would love to see big food, and big pharma, take big hits to their pockets, but it will never happen as long as WE are so greatly outnumbered. If you are with me, gather some allies and fight the resistance. If not, enjoy your supersize fries and soda, but don't get in the way of those of us who want to look and feel great. We care about those around us who want us to be around for a long time — healthy and strong.

11

DON'T BELIEVE
EVERYTHING
YOU THINK...

I always write about how you need to get your mind right to get your body tight, and mindset is the primary function that drives us to either success, keeps us at mediocrity, or leads us to failure. I preach this to you on a fitness level, and other people on a personal 'life' level, that once you have an "I can do" attitude (like when you walk into my gym and work with the guidance of myself and my staff), it's impossible to fail. Well that holds true in every aspect of life, not just fitness. It doesn't matter if you have the best trainer or coaches in the world (my clients do), or if you have access to the most expensive and latest equipment around, if your mind isn't in the game, your outcome will not be ideal.

I know this holds true on a business level also. I compare my own business to my clients and what they are going through with their own health and fitness programs. I have a coach who keeps me accountable just like they do. I needed to seek the help of business experts, because this was all new and intimidating to me when I started, and today, I still seek help of experts. When I see my coaches, they help me with my mindset, and tell me that if I follow what they are telling me to do, and do it with confidence, it is impossible for me to fail.

Last weekend I attended a business mastermind meeting with about 60 other Fit Body Boot Camp Owners, as well as the head brass, including the owner of the company. When I got on that plane, I wasn't in a good place. My business was doing great, my clients were all getting amazing results, and I was feeling strong physically, but my mind wasn't right. And I couldn't understand why.

<u>Strength in numbers</u>

When it came time for me to speak at the round table, I confessed for the first time that I was struggling. I felt disorganized, and that anxiety and stress were crippling me from taking my next step to success. I had no reason for it, as I mentioned above. On paper everything looked great, but in my head, things were wrong. Mind trash was getting to me. But despite all this, I got up every day and fought through it because I refuse to fail and be a victim. I wasn't on the verge of failure, but staying the same or being mediocre isn't an option for me either, and I hadn't grown financially in a couple of months. Well it seemed a lot of others were going through almost the same pressures and stress that life dishes out, some even worse. But we all talked and offered solutions to each other, and I felt better after the discussion.

At lunch, I went into the hallway and had a private heart to heart conversation with the founder of the corporation, and he confessed to me that on occasion, he too suffered from stress and anxiety. What? My mentor? The guy I look up to coach me to success? The guy responsible for making hundreds of people successful has issues with stress? I thought this guy was bionic. Suddenly I started feeling a sense of relief — I wasn't alone. I was around people, including a powerful influential leader, who were in the same situation and feeling the same pressures I was.

I know that many people who I'm working with to obtain their fitness goals are suffering from the same issues. Without addressing the "mental trash" that follows them, which we do every day (and isn't found in many gyms where it's in and out and you're on your own) they couldn't push beyond and reach their goals. There's strength in numbers, and being around positive support works. It makes you feel human, and when you see other people succeeding, it makes you want to push harder to do the same. You know the term "misery loves company?" Well, so does success. And when you surround yourself with like-minded people who are willing to give you a hand, and pick you up off the canvas, your chances of success are more likely. And that's how we roll. Family and friends are always there for us, but it's not the same as being in the company of people with the same goals and struggles.

Cleaning out the mind trash

The following week, I read one and a half books, changed my mind-set, started waking up earlier, and got organized at work. It felt like a weight had been lifted off my chest. Will I still get stressed out on occasion? Yes. Will I still feel anxious until I am where I want to be? Yes. But now I can put things in perspective, realize I am human, and accept that it's all part of this thing called life.

Know that no matter what struggles you face, you are not alone. There are people around you who are experiencing the same or even worse. We are all human, and everyone will need some help on some level in their lives. It's helpful to know that even the people we look up to, and seek guidance from, have been where we are and understand. Also know that whatever your situation is or how bad it gets, everything is solvable. Never quit striving to achieve your goals. They are there to be crushed, and once your mind is right, you will succeed.

12

TIME PASSAGES

W hen did you discover you were out of shape, unhealthy, or unfit? When did this happen? Why did this happen? And if you could turn back the hands of time, what would you do differently? I was watching a show on television this week, and every time someone got shot or died, time would be rewound to get a more favorable outcome. I started thinking… most of us weren't born fat, out of shape, diabetic or with high cholesterol. We were born healthy, didn't need to be taught how to roll, crawl, stand up or walk; yet many people find these simple tasks difficult. What is happening to the human population, and why are simple infant developmental movements so difficult for many to do?

Think back

When did this happen to you? Were you heavy as an adolescent and it stayed with you until now? Were you a lazy teenager who kept getting worse into adulthood? Did it start after college, marriage, childbirth, or in retirement? Think about it long and hard, and try to remember when you were last able to perform movements effortlessly. Can you remember the time when you walked up a flight of stairs without being out of breath, or fit into your skinny jeans and actually liked the way you looked? The bad news is that we can't reboot the system and go back in time to get to the place we once were, but we can look ahead and get back there… in the future.

The past is the past

It drives me crazy when people tell me they were in great shape when they were younger, or were great athletes in college, or how thin they were before giving birth. I always tell them they can get back there with a little hard work and effort. Let's face it folks, you need to get out of the mindset that you are what you are and accept it as the forever you. Stop thinking that you can't get back to where you were — because you can. I have a guarantee for my clients at Fit Body Boot Camp that says if they follow my advice and my program, they will get the results they want. No other fitness facility can guarantee that. I do it because I know without a doubt that everybody has the capability to be their best. It isn't easy, and it takes proper planning, hard work, and a lot of discipline, but it can be done.

We all know somebody with a success story. A woman gives birth, and three months later she is doing a fitness contest. Or an obese guy from high school who cleaned up his act and looks better than when he was younger. Or the grandmother who still bikes, gardens, and lives a vital life. Why can these people achieve results, live a healthy lifestyle, and still look great? Because they give it thought, effort, and they don't jump on quick fixes and harmful things that give them instant gratification. They eat the grilled chicken instead of the chicken parm. They eat baked, not mashed potatoes. They broil fish instead of frying. They walk up the stairs, don't wait for the closest parking space, and they hike while others are watching TV.

Choices you make

You see, it's all about the choices you make that determine the outcome of your health. You need to be ready and decide that you need to make a change. It is at that time, when you decide you have had enough, and you put a plan into action, that you will begin to show results. I was talking with a client and they said how simple it is to get fit and feel great again. Simple, yes, but not easy. Nothing worth anything is easy, but the formula is simple. Eat real unprocessed food, exercise regularly, drink lots of water, and get plenty of rest. That's it. It takes planning and some effort on your part but it can be done, and has been done, by many. If you are unsure or nervous about getting started, give a pro a call. I can put you on a program and you will be feeling better within a week's time. Guaranteed. So think back to where you were before you started your steady decline, and picture yourself back there again, because it is possible. The only thing stopping you from getting there is YOU.

13

Everything Old
Is New Again

E volve or die. Embrace change and don't be afraid of it. Times are changing and so must you. Stop being a dinosaur and get with the times. These are sayings that the younger more tech savvy people are saying to the older generation regarding this constantly changing environment we live in, and I have to agree with the terminology to a certain extent. I believe when it comes to business, and certain conveniences in life, we need to make changes in order to survive and be productive. For instance in business, advertising in the Yellow Pages might no longer be the best avenue to increase your revenue, and when you travel, having GPS navigation is a lot more efficient than carrying around a fold-up map. At home, a programmable thermostat is not only a nice feature, it's almost a must for energy conservation. Email has replaced "snail mail" in all areas of our lives. Communication is expected to be instantaneous.

All these things are changes for the better, however, there is one thing that plays an important part in our lives that is suffering because of these updates and changes that reflect our need for convenience and "new." And that's the way we take care of our health. With all the fast food / quick fixes and fast-acting products out there, we have actually gone backward in the way we take care of ourselves. Rather than being preventative in our self-care in order to prevent disease, we have become a very reactive culture. Instead of doing what is right and healthy now, we wait until we are sick or overweight before we take action.

What can we learn about our health today, from 100 years ago?

I have known about and preached against this for many years, but what has opened my eyes even wider and helped me realize how backward we have become, is an old book a friend gave me from his yard sale. The book was written in the 1920s. It was written by someone named Winslow and the name of the book is *Healthy Living*. How interesting it was to read things like this — from the 1920s: *"A boy learned to ride, swim, climb, and jump from the age of seven on. He trained himself to bear the heavy weight of the suits of armor which the knights wore in battle."* (No, he didn't spend his time in front of videos games and television all summer, way back then.) *"Health and strength, come largely from habits of healthy living, in order to form such habits, you must know something about your body and how it works and what you can do to make it stronger."* (And in this day and age we know!!)

"When we wake [up], the body should be made ready for the work of the day by waking to a few simple exercises. You will find if you do this that you will grow stronger all the time, and better able to play games and run and jump and climb, and you will find yourself happier and more full of life and energy in everything you do" (Hey, pretty amazing... that still works.)

"Sometimes a child will skip breakfast. This is a very bad plan indeed, for soon that child will begin to have an empty feeling inside, he will become cross and fretful and will be stupid in school and work and weak at play. Remember, the body needs plenty of food, and no child can be very much use to himself or anyone else unless he has started off the morning with a good breakfast." (Even in 1920, kids performed better with breakfast.)

Some old advice

This book goes on and on giving validation to most of what I pre-scribe to be healthy. It even goes as far as to say that sunlight and fresh air are good for us. It is all plain and simple folks: eat properly, move functionally, and get proper rest. It is the one prescription that doesn't have an expiration date, because time doesn't diminish the potency of a healthy lifestyle, it enhances it.

So, my suggestion is to keep going to modernize and keep up with the times — increase your social networks to 10,000 fans, keep up-dating to more useful cell phones, iPads, and such. Let's work on our technology so we can send people from 200 miles beneath the ocean to Mars and back. But let's also take what we know still works from the past. And while we're at it, eliminate what science is telling us about a lot of the new things in our lives — get rid of the drive-thru fast food, go back to paper, kick the Styrofoam and plastic... And while I'm at it, let me say this — stop making and using recumbent bicycles, or ab machines, or "get ripped quick" books. It's an old-school statement: "if it ain't broke don't fix it." Or, pick up a health book from the 20s — you could be shocked at how revolutionary all those "old" concepts can sound.

14

FAIL TO PLAN?
PLAN TO FAIL.

Over the past 20 years, I have attended continuing education courses that pertain to exercise, human function, movement patterns, and holistic nutrition. I have gained a ton of knowledge over this time, and I still continue to educate myself, but lately, I have been attending courses that will help me market myself and try to earn my potential based on my level of expertise. The one thing both these methods of education have taught me is that in order to be successful at anything, you need to prioritize and put the important elements of your goal first.

There are many factors and moving parts to whatever it is you try to accomplish, whether it be building your business, raising a family, or trying to get fit and healthy. In order to utilize your time efficiently, and succeed, you have to make a list and prioritize the most important elements of this list, because time is limited. For this article, I will give you examples of things related to health and fitness. (I am not very knowledgeable at the other two — but I am working hard on the business plan part....)

Nutrition first

The number one priority in your quest for health and fitness must be your nutrition plan. Without sound nutrition, you will fail to become healthy. You can get fit "looking" by eating low-fat artificial food and manmade supplements, but my goal is overall health, and you can't become and maintain good health by doing so. Make food quality priority one. Now to take it a step further, if you find yourself wondering what types of food to eat, make protein your priority, especially if you train hard. Protein will help build and repair muscle tissue, and it will take fewer calories to satisfy you, keeping you strong and lean. I always advise balanced nutrition, but if you are pinched for time, or low on funds, make protein a priority.

Balance & core strength

When you begin an exercise program, your number one priority needs to be balance and core strength. If not, it's like trying to build a house on a sand bank. It may stand for a while, but eventually, the foundation will erode and it will come crashing down. Do not load the body unless your foundation is strong and balanced enough. If you currently go to the gym, strength training should be first on this list. And if time is limited, it should be done before cardio vascular exercises. There are great reasons for this: it builds muscle, and muscle burns even more calories at rest, and with proper strength training, your posture will improve and your chance of injury will decrease. You can make it metabolic by performing super sets or doing time intervals with little rest between sets, thus improving your heart and lung strength. When time becomes a factor, and you need to prioritize exercises, then squats, dead lifts, shoulder presses, and a rotational exercise will cover all the essentials: strength, mobility, and stability — creating balance throughout the body.

If you fail to plan, then you should plan to fail. This line has been following me around for years, and I have proven this to myself many times. One example of this was not getting to the market and to buy healthy snacks before a road trip. This should have been a priority equal to getting fuel. Instead, I thought I could wing it and grab something where I was going, only to discover a town with fast food and dollar stores on every corner. I settled for beef jerky and mass-produced yogurt from a convenience store. No plan equals failed nutrition. So let this line play in your head, make a list, and highlight the important stuff. Plan and prioritize, and you will prevail.

15

FEEL INVINCIBLE

The best part of my profession is knowing that what I do promotes positivity, health, and a sense of mental wellness. I take people to their physical limits by constantly reassuring them that what they are doing is going to pay big dividends in the long run. When you work with me you get more than a beat down and long bouts of muscle aches. You see, my intentions are not to make you vomit and pass out (that's easy), but to actually make you feel better about yourself when you walk out the door. I am not here to make you feel inferior, but to take your self-esteem to new levels, by having you do things you thought weren't possible.

One mouthful at a time

I know that working out, by itself, isn't going to take you to new levels of fitness unless you clean up your nutrition plan. I always start by recommending you take small steps and progress until you can reach optimal results. Progressions are the key to success, because most people are reluctant to make even small changes, let alone huge lifestyle overhauls all at once. One example of a dietary change would be to cut out high glycemic foods, such as processed carbohydrates, or inflammatory foods such as pasteurized dairy. Once you change a few habits, and start to see and feel the results, it gets easier from then on.

Get out of the gym

An easy way to start a fitness program is to find something you like doing that will expend energy — something that will be more fun than just lifting weights, and not boring like walking on a treadmill. Some examples would be to run on the beach, hike in the woods, swim, or play tennis. Once you get into a regular practice of moving, then you can start hitting the gym for bigger results with more intensity. Better yet, find something you like but take it to the next level, and bring out your inner beast. This is the type of activity that will not only get you stronger and leaner, because you need to train for it, but it will have you pounding on your chest when you complete the activity. Some examples are: a mud run, a 5k or some obstacle course race, a volleyball tournament, or playing in a tennis or racquetball league. Hey — you can join my fit body boot camp, which will give you that feeling of being part of a team, give you fun and exciting workouts, and net you results, guaranteed.

Mind and body

The special interest that brings out the beast in me is mountain biking. When you are going downhill at ridiculous rates of speed, knowing that one wrong move means disaster, you feel it. When you climb a steep hill, and your legs and lungs are feeling like they are going to explode, you feel it. This feeling makes you want to push harder, get stronger, and never quit wanting to do it because your adrenaline is pumping so hard that your endorphins make you feel invincible. You will get this feeling from competitive activities as well. Whatever it takes to get you moving, you need to jump at the opportunity. Hire a trainer, hike, walk on the beach, or compete in an event. Do whatever it takes to create a new and improved you; be more fit, happier and more productive in everyday life.

16

GET A BETTER BOTTOM... *LINE*

In spring people who are cooped up in offices can be seen with their suit and sneakers at lunchtime, or, if they're really lucky, in the company gym. If there's time they can sneak out to go to their own gym and rush back. Companies are also realizing that the fitness of their employees reduces their spiraling healthcare costs. So, it makes good business sense to help your employees stay well. That doesn't mean taking a leisurely stroll around the block then having that pizza delivery for lunch. Want to have a healthy workforce? Have a healthier workplace! Here are some tips on how to do just that.

It starts at the top

For wellness campaigns to be successful in the workplace, the commitment and participation from company leadership goes a long way to long term acceptance from employees. Leading by example is key — from the top, down. Preferably the CEO will want to show her/his buy-in by participating in activities, issuing incentives, and providing recognition, too.

Healthy food zone

When you walk into work in the morning, do you see doughnuts and muffins in the break room? Maybe there is some leftover pizza from yesterday's quick meeting? If you have vending machines, take an inventory — what is being offered? (Hint: fat filled granola bars and yogurt with high sugar content is not healthy.) Most vending companies offer healthy alternatives — so take a look, make requests to management, and watch those healthy changes happen. How about a purified water source? That can be a water filter or a free-standing supplier. Get rid of the soda and juice machines. I believe banning foods can create a backlash of defiance; so lead with the carrot (pun intended), not the stick.

Fitness programs

Next, is there a room where you can exercise? You can recruit someone to lead classes on a regular basis. Even popping in an exercise or yoga tape is better than nothing. If you can't work out during work hours, then build some hoopla about meeting right after work. Of course, the ideal that I'd like to see is employees who get help with their membership to a gym — like mine at Providence Fit Body Boot Camp. Employees consistently say, when surveyed, that their pay is not the number one thing that makes them happy at work — it's often how the company values them with extras such as a fitness opportunity. Bring it up at employee benefit time. Or, talk to your company's health insurer to see if partial compensation is available for gym memberships.

Incentives and Recognition

If you can't pay part of employees' fitness programs, offer incentives for accomplishments — a cash incentive, a parking place, or gift certificates for local businesses, and don't forget to show that important recognition before fellow employees. Wellness campaigns help employees jump start their own fitness and health programs — and they also help employers have strong, cohesive, and happy teams of employees. Make it fun! You'll reap the rewards.

Let's Review

Encouraging wellness is good business. You will have a happier workforce. You may also be able to reduce absenteeism and save on health insurance. Your employees will be stronger and less likely to suffer injuries like when moving a heavy box, or physical labor jobs. Your employees will value this, and you will be able to retain good employees. It is costly for a company to hire and re-train.

While focusing on exercise, don't forget that 80 percent of any wellness program is the food you eat. By making your company a healthy environment, it will show to others when you have meetings and visitors. Working as a team at work means you will be a better team — at work. Everyone gets to be part of the team — young and older employees alike. Group events also help to eliminate troublesome cliques at work. Finally, the concept of doing well by doing good is real. Your company will be more successful. While that's not a promise, it is something I see all the time. Successful workplace health programs have shown us what is possible — we just need to dig deeper as employers and make it happen. Need help? Give me a call. Your bottom line could look a whole lot better.

17

FIT FOR LIFE — YES, YOU CAN!

I was at a networking event for one of my clients, and I was talking to an individual who seemed to have no interest in taking care of herself. I was describing some of my programs and fitness challenges that I run at my facility, and every response from her contained some sort of sarcastic negative remark. Of course, I was more and more irritated as she spoke. I was explaining how I give cash rewards for the person that does the most pushups, and she asked if I also give prizes for the least amount, because that would be the contest she would enter. I then said no, but if you can't do too many in the beginning, you could still win money because I give prizes for to the person that improves the most and has the biggest increase in the number they can do. I told her that everyone in my program improves with these challenges, and she kept joking about how she would be the one that did the least. I kept insisting that everyone improves, and she kept telling me how hopeless she was, followed by laughter and bites of pizza (as she had a comical attitude about her admitted terrible diet).

After three minutes of trying to convince her that if she wanted to, she could be fit and healthy, I moved on and started talking to another business professional who kept rubbing his gut and asking if there was any hope for a guy who loves beer and ribs. Needless to say, I didn't stay at that event too long. Approximately 20 minutes later I was on my way home. I understand that health and fitness doesn't appeal to everyone, nor does hard work, sacrifice and discipline, but even if self-improvement isn't something you care about, then why do make a mockery of it?

Why is it that sometimes people who care about themselves, workout regularly, and eat healthy foods, get treated like outcasts? Look around and take note of what our population looks like. About 37 percent of Americans are obese, so that leaves 63 percent who are not considered obese. But out of that percentage, how many are actually in GOOD shape? Maybe 10 percent? When you look at the distribution of wealth in this country, and notice that only a small percentage of people are truly wealthy, do you make fun of them, and joke about how hard they worked to get to their position in life? Why would anyone criticize someone for doing something positive for themselves? Am I a pain because I choose not to eat GMOs and ask wait staff in a restaurant what is in my food or where the food comes from, or how it is prepared?

What have we become? Heck, there are even gym chains that encourage this by giving pizza, bagels, and candy to their clients. Are we just accepting that it's part of a normal existence to follow the masses and destroy ourselves day by day, and to chastise the ones who are fighting the resistance, and actually care about themselves? This bothers me because I take what I do very seriously. I know how good it feels to wake up every day and know that I am on top of my game, and every day I am going to improve some aspect of my life in some way.

How do you see yourself?

When you wake up and look at an overweight individual in the mirror, is it difficult for you to have a strong sense of self-respect? If you don't care about yourself, or aren't proud of yourself, then you aren't going to care about other things in your life as you should — like your career or other things around you. Maybe that's why people attempt to bring down others who are their opposites.

This is why I do what I do for a living, because I want to change as many lives as I can. I feel that once you start to care about yourself, your whole demeanor changes, and you become a more positive person, and it starts to rub off on others.

It is a nice feeling when I finish a session and everyone gives each other a high five and says, "great job." Positivity is contagious, and you need to surround yourself with like-minded people in order to succeed at anything you do. I heard a story at a business seminar about a guy walking the beach, and he stumbles upon a fisherman with a bucket of crabs. As he observes the crabs in the bucket, he notices one trying to escape. He informs the fisherman that one is getting away, and the guy just tells him to sit and watch what happens. As the crab is about to get to the rim of the bucket, other crabs reach up and pull him back in. This seems to be the way humans react to others that are doing something better and more positive than they are. They just reach up and try to pull others back to their level.

We've got this — together

This is why I am creating a community of positive people who are trying to get their health and fitness together and are serious about doing it. I never allow negative energy to exist in my place, and I even reprimand someone for saying "I can't." The term I make them use is "this is tough for me, but I will try harder until I get better at it." This holds true with everything in life from business to fitness. You have a better chance of becoming successful when you surround yourself with positive like-minded people. Have you ever noticed that negative people find a problem for every solution? If you want success in any part of your life, you need to turn your back on the crabs, and keep moving forward and working hard to achieve your goals. If it is health and fitness you want, give me a call, and we can do this together.

18

GET A COACH. I DID.

INSANITY (def): extreme foolishness or irrationality. This is the original definition, (but I like the Albert Einstein version) doing the same thing over and over again and expecting different results.

Regardless of how you read the definition, if you work out day after day, sweat gallons a week, wake up sore, tired and fatigued, and can't see changes in your physique, then what you are doing might meet that definition of insanity. If you invest time and effort into doing ANYTHING, you should see results fairy quickly and often. I don't care if it is building a business, career, house, or your body. If you invest time and true effort and aren't seeing favorable results, it's time to make a change — NOW. I used to see it every day at the gym. Month after month, the same people would lumber in, get on the same machine, work out at the same intensity, and look the same or worse. Or I would see the gym maniacs go charging in, jump on a piece of cardio equipment, go like a bat out of hell for hours, and still look the same day after day, week after week. I would sometimes go up to certain people, and say, "Hey, I noticed how hard you work, are you happy with the results you are getting?" Most times I would hear "No, and I don't understand why." That's when I would offer my input, and usually

49

get a big eye-opening response from the individual. And, frequently, I would acquire a new client.

So why do we do this to ourselves?

If you own a business, and you keep dumping all your money and investing all your time into making it profitable and you still lose money every year, wouldn't you realize that what you are doing is wrong and make a change? Or would you keep going until you go bankrupt? Sadly, sometimes the answer is "yes" to both questions. I don't know "why" but I have a remedy to fix the negative outcome — HIRE A COACH. Put your ego on a shelf and realize you can't be good at everything. When you enter a field or take on a certain task that you are not completely knowledgeable about, you need to seek guidance. No this is not the easy way out, but it is the smart way. I like to look at it as the most efficient way to do things too, because our time is our most valuable resource. Once it's spent, it's gone. There are no refunds, and we all get the same limited number — 24 hours a day. So why waste it?

5 Things a GOOD coach will do for you

1. Motivate you to be the best you can be, by pushing you out of your comfort zone.

2. Protect you from harm, by knowing the proper precautions to take.

3. Hold you accountable for your actions, by pushing you and not letting you make excuses.

4. Make it difficult for you to fail by being knowledgeable and experienced in their field.

5. Give you direction, and put you on the path to productivity that will prevent you from wasting time.

I have been coaching people for the past 20 years, helping them reach their health and fitness goals. When you work out with me you'll get inspirational coaching, using all the steps I have mentioned above. By doing so you will eliminate all the guesswork associated with fitness, and be able to reach your goal in the safest and most efficient way possible. But while I think I'm the best of the best in coaching people about health and fitness, I knew that when it came to business and systems, I was just as much in need of that type of coach. So, I did my research and chose to go with a large national franchise that I could bring to Rhode Island, with its best practices already in place, so I could focus on doing what I was best at — working with my clients. I have a coaching staff that is accessible and helps motivate me and gives me business direction. Without this, I could waste serious amounts of time and money by guessing or using trial and error tactics. I have neither time nor money to waste, so I am trusting my coaching staff to help me through my journey.

Find the right coach

By finding the right coach, I've gained great insight, direction and motivation that is giving me the confidence to live my dream, and reach my goals of helping hundreds of people reach theirs. By making changes, and keeping my mind and eyes open, I feel I have gained more business and marketing sense in the last 6 months than I have in the past 20 years. I know the value of coaching for attaining maximal fitness even more now too, so my best piece of fitness advice to you is to hire a coach to guide you through your journey, be coachable, quit wasting time, and stop the insanity. Do this and you, too, will be fired up and motivated to reach your destination.

19

GET RID OF
YOUR F.E.A.R.

*T*his is hard. I have trouble with that. I am not very good at doing this. That isn't my strong point.

I hear these lines all the time at my facility, and my response is always the same. Good, now that we have exposed your weaknesses, let's go after them, and make them disappear.

I have a philosophy that when something you do troubles you, you should attack it rather than avoid it. Many people have the wrong attitude when they face adversity; they tend to ignore the situation rather than shine a brighter light on it. If you do this, you will never get better or advance, and the problem will never go away. If you can't do a pushup when you come in here, don't tell me you can't do pushups, because you can — maybe just not right now, but you will. And saying "I can't" just affirms that you never will. If others are doing it, you can, too. I will make modifications and show you some alternative actions that will help you progress until you can do it. If you have an injury, that's another story. That's a legitimate reason, and you shouldn't attempt any action that will bring you further injury or pain. But if a task is giving you trouble only because it's difficult for you to do, I say to roll up your sleeves, and let's conquer it.

This philosophy doesn't just apply to physical fitness and exercise, it can be used academically, socially, and in business, too. If you are going to school, and math isn't your strong point, what should you do? You can't avoid the subject, so you either need to hire a tutor and get extra help, or spend more time finding a way to get better. That's it. Don't ignore. Just try harder, take a different approach, and you will get better at whatever it is you want to be doing.

If you feel socially awkward being around people, you need to get out more, and attend more social events. After a while, being around people will be no big deal. I am terrible with technology, so I try to spend more time getting better at it. I also make regular trips to the Apple store to get help for my questions. I know I will never be great because I don't invest enough time into it to be great, but I can do enough, and do what I need to do to be accomplished.

F.E.A.R — False Evidence Appearing Real

This is what keeps most of us from achieving our goals and accomplishing our dreams. It's letting some crazy emotion get in our way, and bringing our mindset to a place of failure. What's in your head WILL get in your way. A quote from Henry Ford states that if you believe you can, or if you believe you can't, you are correct in both instances. The more you think like this, the more you will realize that most of what will either move us forward, or pull us back, comes from mindset and what is in our head. False evidence can appear real. Think back about all the things that worried or scared you in the past, everything from monsters under your bed to learning how to drive. When you look back, you think about how ridiculous it was to be afraid of these things. Now look at more recent things that had you scared, but when you got past the initial anxiety, it's now just a normal procedure you execute every day. Moving to a new place, joining a gym, meeting the in-laws, kids going to college… these are all changes that will initially take you out of your comfort zone and cause a little fear, but once you take the initial plunge, it gets easier.

Believe You Can

When I first opened Providence Fit Body Boot Camp, I was nervous as hell, but I attended marketing conferences and business summits, and realized that many other people run successful businesses, so why can't I? Now the fear is just replaced with the stress of running it to perfection, and keeping all my clients happy, which I probably never can, totally, but it motivates me to keep striving for improvement every day. Looking back, I wouldn't change a thing.

So if you are putting off joining a gym (or at least mine) because you are afraid of being judged, or feel you are not good at working out, don't. Get rid of the mind trash and realize that many others have been in your position. And after a few workouts, their confidence rises, and they conquer their workouts. If you are not good at pushups, no worries, we will make sure to help you, until you do them and do them well. Then you'll just feel silly for being afraid of your F.E.A.R.

20

IS YOUR FITNESS PROGRAM MAKING YOU UNFIT?

A healthy body won't get fat — and a poorly nourished body won't get healthy. Stop doing something over and over and not getting results. Losing body fat and gaining muscle while becoming leaner and stronger should be the goal. If you are working out and this isn't happening, it's time to make a change. Time is too valuable to waste, and exercise is too much effort to get results, or not the intended results. If this sounds like where you are in your fitness routine, here are a couple of alternatives to what you are doing which will put you on the road to success.

Nutrition

You put too much of a strangle hold on your nutrition and pay too much attention to calorie counting. My first and most important piece of advice goes to food quality. Get rid of processed cheap food and eat quality whole, organic foods. Because if you focus on counting calories, you end up eating low quality, heavily processed fat free products like fat-free mayo, fat-free yogurt, and other processed fat free dairy products, low-fat butter, oil substitutes, packaged meats, and reduced calorie beverages. You also sacrifice healthy fats by eating egg whites and low-fat peanut butter. Instead, purchase quality organic whole foods, eat yolks and full-fat butter and dairy products (if you need to eat dairy). This type of food is absorbed nutritionally by the body and gets properly utilized and digested, and you will feel more satisfied when you eat less. Remember, your body needs fat and nutrients to function effectively and efficiently, build muscle, and fight disease and sickness, so don't deprive yourself of nutrients.

Once you master the habit of quality eating, you can eliminate certain things and portion your foods accordingly. Usually by this time you will already have lost some weight and will look and feel better.

Overtraining

Overtraining results in a negative outcome in several ways. I see a lot of people spending hours every day exercising on elliptical machines and recumbent bikes and they do not get the results they are looking for. On the contrary, these people usually get flabbier due to the fact they are burning muscle and not building it. Training for longer amounts of time with little intensity nets you poor results. My suggestion would be to cut down on the cardio time and up the intensity level. Hit it harder and shorter. I would rather see someone doing intervals on the treadmill, taking a spin class, or doing a step mill for 30 minutes over walking for an hour on the phone, or watching TV on a stationary bike any day.

Many women worry about getting too big from lifting weights. This is the main reason they neglect strength training. I feel the number one most important part of any exercise program is strength work. For those who work with me, after going through body weight movements, they become stable and move. Everyone I train from 15 to 87 years-old does strength training. Not only does this make you look better and move more effectively, it also revs up your metabolism to make your body burn more calories at rest. The higher your muscle to fat ratio is, the more efficient you become at torching that unwanted body fat. It has also been shown that after a bout of resistance training, you burn calories longer than if you did a session of cardio.

A prescription for success

In this day and age, especially where there is big money to be made selling fitness tapes, equipment, expensive memberships and classes, things are being blown out of proportion as to what it takes to get in shape. Much of what is new is overdone and quite extreme. "Insanity" type programs, px90, CrossFit, and beat down workouts, are in my opinion, a little too much for most people who are lured into what sounds like a quick fix. Everything is extreme to a point that if you don't vomit or get sore for days you are not successful. I believe exercise should be looked at like medication: too much = overdose. Too little = ineffective. Prescribe just the right dose and you will get the results you need.

21

GOT DRIVE?

What separates us as humans? Why are some of us wealthy and some poor? Some fit, some overweight? Some famous, some unknown? I people watch all day long — at the market, Home Depot, high school football games, airports, you name it. Some people watch for fashion, but I am observing posture, movements, body language, and body mass. I understand that some people have medical problems, or flawed genetics, but I believe that what separates most of us is DRIVE. It is a person's amount of drive that will enable them to perform at a certain level. When one has the drive to be fit, they will seek any way possible to learn to do so. When one has the drive to be wealthy, they exert all their time and energy to do so also. This is more likely to produce the desired result. One can argue and say it's because people are uneducated, and don't know how to better themselves, but all the info is out there, it just takes drive to find it.

What is DRIVE, and how do you get it?

D-esire: you need to have this first. You can't pick a task out of a hat and expect to excel at it. If your parents forced you to play sports, and you had no desire to, you would lack internal drive and probably not be very good at it. The same goes for your health; if you have no desire to improve it, you won't.

R-egularity: you won't become a real estate top producer if you only seek listings once in a while. You won't get in the best shape of your life after one workout or one day of eating healthy; you won't be a good hitter if you hit the batting cages once a week. You need regularity, and it takes drive to do something over and over again.

I-ntensity: do something without intensity and the results will be uneventful. Train without intensity and chances are that you will stay the same. Play football without intensity, and your team will lose. It is the people with lackluster attitudes and lack of intensity who usually are not at the top of their game because intensity feeds drive.

V-ision: is a necessary component to all success, because without it, you will have no direction, and without direction, having drive is useless. If you start working out and do not visualize what you want to look like, you probably will lack the intensity and desire to get you there. If you start a construction project without a vision, you will be spending a lot of money on changes until you get it right. Start anything without a vision and you probably won't finish.

E-xecute: when you have all the other components, you are more likely to execute the goal at hand. Without execution, you will have nothing. Thinking about a career move won't make it happen. Talking about opening a business will not put food on the table. Trying to eat better will not get you fit and healthy — doing it will. Everything is talk and thoughts until something is executed and put into play.

So what separates us as humans? Why are some strong and some weak? Why are some followers and some leaders? Why are some employed and some not? What creates different classes in this world, whether it be income or weight?

DRIVE!

22

How Bad Do You Want It?

I keep hearing how busy everyone is, and that they aren't sure if they can fit working out into their schedule. Well, *make it* fit your schedule. Actually, make it part of your schedule. It's very easy to miss workouts, but it's also easy to get them in when you make them part of your schedule.

Delegate a time — 3x per week — and make it work. Providence Fit Body Boot Camp, for instance, runs 9 sessions daily Mon-Fri from 5:25 am until 6:30 pm. So unless you are working 13 hours a day (some do, most don't) you have no excuse not to be in shape, unless it's not that important to you.

At my facility, we have well over 100 people who pass through daily, getting it done. And guess what? Most have careers, kids, families, and dogs to take care of, and they still find a way to get to the gym and take care of themselves.

Time

The whole time thing. Yes, I know we're all busy. Maybe you pick your kids up from school every day. Have you ever told them to take the bus — or even walk home — because you don't have time to pick them up? Most likely you haven't. Have you ever not provided the family dinner because you didn't have time? Maybe you pick up take-out, or make something quick when you have had a busy day, but you still feed everyone, and you get it done.

Why is this? Because there are things we make a priority in life. We do them, they get done. Health and fitness should be no different. Unless you work an incredibly physical job, you need to move and exercise in a planned way. And that is reason enough to make it a priority and make it part of your schedule. Random acts of exercise aren't good enough. You have to be consistent, and embed it into your lifestyle. I see the results daily. The clients that live it, get better results than the ones who are not consistent. Every bit is positive, but when you want outstanding results, you need to devote the time, and be consistent.

I am not an exercise person you say?

Well, just what is that supposed to mean? Exercise is nothing more than movement. We do it at a higher intensity to overload the body, create resistance, and elevate the heart rate. But it's still basic movements we normally perform every day. We need to increase the intensity to achieve results, and push ourselves out of our comfort zone. But the principle is to mimic daily life so you will not only be fit but also more productive. So unless you spend your life living on a sofa, and don't need to do anything or move at all, exercise IS for you.

I can't afford it

I love this excuse. The first thing I say to that is: If you have cable TV, a smart phone, or a vehicle with tons of options, you can afford to join a gym. Cable TV allows you to sit around and do nothing for your body except get lethargic. This is not a necessity in anyone's life, but almost everyone spends a lot of time doing it. And not just a little time and money to get just the basics — news, weather, etc. All those premium stations cost a lot of money, so don't say you can't afford the gym when you have a premium bundle of senseless options on your television. Smart phones cost a bunch too, but if you want one, I guarantee you will find a way to get one whether you can afford it or not.

So all the reasons like time, money, and the fact you don't like to exercise, are just poor excuses that are going to keep you over-weight and unhealthy. It's all about the mindset. Because when you want something bad enough, human nature helps you find a way to go out and get it. So, next time someone asks you why you aren't in shape, just reply, "Because I don't care enough yet about myself to dedicate the time it takes to make improvements in my life." Leave the other excuses on the shelf, and be honest with yourself.

My question to you is this: How bad do you want it?

23

HOW FAR
HAVE YOU COME?

"It's a slow process, but quitting won't speed it up."
~ Unknown

"If you look closely, most overnight success stories were actually a slow process." ~ Steve Jobs

Those are two good quotes to digest, especially if you are like me (impatient) and want things done immediately, or want instant outcomes. When I want something, I want it now, and I usually overstress myself to try and get it. Then I read a quote, article, book, or talk to my business coach and realize that I am overthinking. I just need to keep working hard and being consistent, and the outcomes I am looking for will happen. I have been in this particular business for just over one year but I want to be in the same position as someone with five years' experience. You see, I never compare myself to people doing less than me, only to the ones ahead of me. This keeps me motivated and driven, while helping me realize that success is a process: never peak, the best is yet to come. Let the process begin.

One step at a time

It's kind of ironic that when a client gets off the scale and hasn't lost as much weight as they expected, I am the one trying to rationalize with them and tell them to be patient and keep working hard. It's a process. When you come to Providence Fit Body Boot Camp, you will get results faster than any other program, but it still takes time, and a lot of hard work, and we guarantee outcomes. I tell my clients during their workouts that every rep, every set, and every workout is one step closer to meeting their goals, and as long as you do not sabotage your journey with unhealthy habits after you leave the gym, you will reach your destination. You need to win one battle at a time in order to win the war.

I tell the high school kids who I coach to focus on each play, and play as hard as you can. If you do this over and over, and give your best, victory is guaranteed. The team that works the hardest and wants it most always wins. I compare it to riding a bicycle up a big hill: Keep looking forward, don't stop pedaling, and do NOT look up because it will discourage you if it looks too hard. But then when you reach the top, look back and see how far you have come. Then enjoy the view. It all starts with mindset. You need to get your mind right, have a vision, and be willing to go for the long haul. Successful businesses and perfect bodies will not happen overnight.

Focus. Execution. Time. Discipline.

You need to be mentally prepared, and *focus* on a goal. What is it? Thirty pounds lighter, fit into that little black dress, do more push-ups, visit Graceland, decrease medications, train for a mud run, or just feel better? Next step in the process is to *execute*. I notice when someone comes to the gym regularly, the results come faster than when they are inconsistent. When they realize they need improvement, they mentally develop a plan, and show up to exercise regularly. In addition, they stick to their nutrition plan. Execution = results. But none of them did it overnight, in a week or even a month. It took *time* and *discipline*. The weight came off one pound at a time. Consistency, mental focus and hard work always gets it done. One pedal stroke, one rep, set, and one workout at a time. It's a process, but the results are worth it. And won't it be great when you get to the top of the mountain? Then you can look back and see how far you've come!

24

How to Be Unstoppable

S o you're working out — a lot. And you're watching your progress. But are you seeing it? Regardless of working harder at your fitness program, you want to look for three things that determine if you are getting results. So stop wasting time, money and energy if you aren't: *Losing Fat — Gaining Muscle — and — Feeling Better.*

If you've reached a plateau or haven't gotten there yet, here are three things you can change to be unstoppable in your fitness progress.

Hydrate. Hydrate. Hydrate.

Our bodies function on a cellular level and cells require water. We hit the gym to build muscle, and muscle is composed of millions of cells. We need enzymes to digest food to build muscle, and water aids in digestion and aids the ability for enzymes to travel. In order to be able to move without cramping, our muscles need water. Get the picture? And that just deals with your needs during exercise. Being properly hydrated also prevents headaches and free radical cell damage caused by environmental toxins. Think: the solution for pollution is dilution! Along with that goes aiding your kidneys and bladder during elimination. It is also responsible for shuttling water soluble vitamins to cells, so when you get dehydrated, it is tougher for the body to absorb nutrients. I recommend one half ounce of water for every pound of body weight per day, any less and you are doing yourself a disservice.

Sleep!

Eight hours sleep is not a luxury; it is a necessity for your wellbeing. When you sleep, great things happen to your body as well as your mind and energy levels. Improving cognitive brain function and increasing energy levels creates a huge network of positive attributes for the body. I hear the excuse all the time, "I am too busy to get that much sleep." Do NOT confuse busy with productive, and if you are well rested, you will become much more productive than when you are tired, lethargic and miserable. The proper amount of sleep will allow you to wake happier and be more energetic. Proper rest allows your mind to wake with clarity. When you have the right mindset from the beginning of the day you accomplish many more tasks and are able to focus more efficiently. When you get the proper amount of sleep, you wake up on fire and are ready to go. Many people think that they are building muscle in the gym. Sorry, but that theory is wrong. When you work out you are actually breaking the body down. Training causes micro tears in the muscle, and the only way to recover from this is with proper sleep and nutrition. If this is not achieved, then you will not recover from physical activity, making positive gains and results nearly impossible.

Eat quality food — frequently — all day long

Not eating quality food is probably the biggest reason you don't get the results you want. When you eat efficiently you will get results faster and achieve your goals. When you consume garbage — processed food — you cause inflammation in the body. Our defense systems prioritize and fight off the most damaging invaders first. This means when you are sick you shouldn't work out because our immune systems are fighting sickness and breaking the body down, causing the immune system to work too hard, prolonging all ailments in the body. So, when you eat badly, the body is too busy fighting inflammation and is too drained to build, repair and do the positive things our bodies need to get results. When you eat quality food, your system works smoothly and efficiently allowing the body to uptake nutrients effectively, thus triggering results and progress.

Want to be Unstoppable?

Let's review… drink lots of clean water… get to bed on time… eat quality food throughout the day… then check your progress. Remember, it's not about how often you do these things or how well you keep to your workout program. It's about three things. Are you losing fat? Gaining muscle? Feeling better? If not, stop doing what you are doing. Talk to your personal trainer — or get one. Your personal trainer should be talking about things beyond weight training. Because YOU want results that will make you — *Unstoppable.*

25

How's That *Resolution* Working for You?

How did that New Year's resolution work out for you this year? If you're reading this, then maybe you made one about losing weight, or exercising more, or getting healthier. Has it happened? Did you get there? Did you change your unhealthy habits and replace them with healthy ones? Did you quit smoking? Lose 50 pounds? Improve your situation in any way, shape, or form?

Now what?

Are you in the best shape of your life? I didn't think so. Now what? I'll tell you "now, what!" If you are like most people, you are going to look for another future date to get "started" on your delusional program. You will play it over and over in your head about how you are going to do it this time, but when the day comes, you will put it off again. You will start thinking about "next" year and how great you are going to be, but that day will probably never come either.

What you need to do is — take action now!!

It drives me crazy when someone calls my gym inquiring about one of my programs on a Wednesday, then tells me they will start on Monday. I always ask, why wait till Monday? You could have completed three workouts by then and be three steps closer to your goal. After giving a few reasons why starting now would be more beneficial, they usually agree and come in the next day. I do this because I know that when people put things off, they usually never get it done. That's why it is important to take immediate action and be persistent when you have a task you need to accomplish. Whether it be a project around the house, vying for a promotion at work, taking a vacation, or getting fit, action takers get the results, and the draggers get nowhere.

So which one are you? If you are the latter and fitness is your goal, put your fears and procrastinating mind at ease. I have a solution for you, and if you take immediate action, and are willing to supply some discipline, you still have time to get more fit before summer. But you have to take action now. Today. I can immediately get you into one of my programs that guarantee fitness and fat loss. The reason why my program will work for you, as it has others, is that I provide structure and make you accountable for your actions.

What is it that keeps us from our goals?

Is it the time commitment? It shouldn't be. Research has shown us that all you need from an exercise program is 30 minutes of intense exercise sessions, three to five days per week, to get you great results.

Or is it fear of failure that's holding you back? Maybe you feel you are not capable, or worthy but that is false, and I know you know that, too. We all have the ability and the right to health and fitness, and you're no different.

Is it bad habits that we can't break? Whatever it is you can fix it, and if you can't fix it, then the problem is in the mirror. It's you and your lack of drive, motivation and discipline. Most of us want perfect health and the most perfect looking body we can get, so why do some achieve it and some don't? Because many of us wait too long and don't take immediate action. Those who do get it done and those who wait, don't. If that is the case, then you need to find a trained professional who will help you not only with exercise, but with the mind games you play with yourself — a great coach to help you succeed.

It starts with now

Waiting for tomorrow isn't the answer. Now is, and always will be the time to get started making positive changes in your life... in whatever area you need to change. Now is the time to get on the fast track to success. So what are you waiting for? Get up off your butt, take a deep breath, and call me — I'll help you put together a plan of action — today. Let's do it.

26

I Don't Want to Hear It... So Don't Say It.

I can't... I'm waiting for... But... I AM trying... After... I should've...

I have found that over the years, the only way to get things done and accomplish anything is to take action and physically do the task that needs to be done. Unless you have the capacity to delegate to others, you have to take action yourself. Thinking about it and gathering good ideas isn't enough. When it comes to health and fitness, you need to take the initiative, get moving and start eating properly. You can't have someone else do it for you.

Even those who hire a professional like me still have to provide some drive, desire, and discipline. This seems to be the hardest part for most people to maintain. First you need to realize that you have a problem before you pick up the phone to call a trainer. Some examples of fitness problems would include an inability to lose weight, tightness, bad posture, or just the need for a kick in the butt to increase intensity. When you do that, you have taken the first step.

Next I will assure you, and even guarantee that you will get the results you want IF you follow my lead. But there are lots of steps to success, and sometimes life gets in the way. And even though you know what it will take to get there, we encounter distractions and psychological roadblocks that slow our process. By changing a few habits and eliminating some negative thoughts, you will find it to be an effective way to accomplish your goals.

Lose the excuses and get back on the path to success!

1. "I can't"

This is the biggest cop-out that you can say to yourself. Whenever there is a task that you think you can't accomplish, ask yourself if others did it, why can't you? My philosophy is that when someone does something that you think you can't do it's because they wanted it more, not because they are better than you. So, if you want something in life like health or wealth, you need to develop an "I can" attitude and go after it.

2. "But I *am* trying"

This is just another way of saying I am not succeeding at something. I am trying to lose weight, or I am trying to find a job. There are many ways to lose weight, and there is always someone hiring. If you are truly trying, you will be saying, "I am doing," because when you give something a true all-out effort, you will achieve your goal and the phrase "I'm trying," won't need to be said. (Exception: I am trying to set a world speed record but I keep coming up seconds short. OK, if you are doing that you can say "I'm trying.")

3. "I am waiting for / after"

For what? You can't wait. And "after" what, and why? Here's a thought — how about now? I will start "after"… my kids are in school/the first of the year/my friends' wedding/the summer. Why can't you get started now, then you will have a head start to whenever "after" will occur? "I am waiting" for someone to call me back/until my friend can join me/to hear back from an employer /until I can join a gym. Do not wait on anyone or anything. This is just a procrastination technique. There is no perfect time. If you are waiting for something that's important to you, you will either follow up or get started on your own. Human nature proves that when we want something bad enough we act, not wait. Lose the phrase "I am waiting," from your vocabulary, and you will be surprised how fast you can move forward when you are not standing around — just waiting.

27

I'VE GOT TWO WORDS FOR YOU

Today I give you two words that will equal success in every area of your life. Whether you are trying to build a house, family, business, or the perfect body, two words come to mind. Without them you will not succeed. You will not succeed because it's nearly impossible to accomplish anything without implementing what these two words stand for, because success and luck don't just happen to people — they are *created* by people. But to create luck and success, you need to abide by the ritual of two unglamorous words: "HARD WORK." I see it around me, and I live it daily.

Are you on the "A" List?

At Providence Fit Body Boot Camp, as well as at every other gym in the world, there are primarily two types of clientele. In my gym, there are those who hang on every word that I say, and do everything I tell them to do. They show up 3 to 5 times per week, and everyone who shows up has to work hard, and then they leave and eat the way they are supposed to eat. Not an easy task to accomplish, but with a work ethic instilled, it's not impossible. These are the clients who are getting amazing results. They exert the extra effort to make time to exercise, and prepare their meals. They don't make excuses, and the words "I can't," are eliminated from their vocabulary. They understand what it takes, and they do whatever it takes to get it done. And the results are always favorable!

Or the "B" List?

The other type of client (and you know who you are) sometimes forgets what it takes, and needs me to remind them on a regular basis to step up their game, and that's OK because that's what I'm here for. They can be inconsistent with their workouts or nutrition program, and that's why progress halts and sometimes even goes backwards. No, I am not picking on my clients, just telling it like it is because everyone knows when they've been focused and working hard or just coasting and going through the motions. You know whether you are cheating with your eating and missing workouts, and I will know if someone is putting in the effort when I ask them to check-in on the scale. The food slackers usually refuse, or confess to doing something detrimental to their health, so I tell them to pick up the pace and clean up their eating for the next few days and I'll get their weight then.

If someone is not getting the results they envisioned, they are not usually surprised and almost always admit they haven't been focused or putting in the effort. I make it clear at my initial consultation that I can create a simple efficient path to their goals, but it won't be easy. It will take a lot of hard work, discipline, and consistency to pull it off. Then I ask them if they are ready for me to hold them accountable for their actions, and get on their case if they don't get results. So, they know if they don't put in the work, I will know at weigh-in time.

I also noticed how the words "hard work" have an impact on the business world. I know many successful and many unsuccessful people, and what separates the two types of people is mindset and work ethic. Everyone has ideas, and envisions themselves in a better place, but what creates the difference is that some are action takers and some refuse to push themselves to put in the hard work required they need to accomplish their goals. Everyone I know who is successful worked their behinds off to get there, and everyone who is not has some excuse, or blames someone else. Yeah, I know some people born into wealth have a leg up, and easier lives, but in order to *build* success, it requires a mindset and "no quit" attitude many don't have.

The choice is yours...

You need to be at work before most are awake, and still be there when most are asleep. You need to work holidays and weekends, and accept that there really won't be such a thing as vacation time, sick days, and 40-hour work weeks. To be truly successful takes more work than the "average" person is willing to put in. Successful lazy people? They rarely exist. The choice is ultimately up to you, and how you want to live your life. Do you want ultimate health and fitness? Do you want to succeed in business? If your answer is "yes," then I am telling you that it's all possible, BUT, only if you are willing to incorporate HARD WORK into your daily routine. If you aren't willing to put in the effort, then you can expect to be "average" at best, on every level of your life. For some of us, that's just not an option.

28

IT STARTS WITH "I CAN"

*T*his is tough! But it's hard! I'm tired! That's heavy! These are all things I hear constantly throughout the day, and it's all part of the program. If people weren't saying these things, I wouldn't be doing my job properly, so I just make a counter remark and keep 'em moving. But the one line I hear regularly, that I jump all over people for saying is "I *can't* do it." Unless someone asks you to lift a tractor or invent a magic pill that will save the world, you should lose this phrase from your vocabulary.

Where would Apple be if Steve Jobs listened to people who told him he would never compete with Microsoft? Or Arnold Schwarzenegger if he listened to people tell him that an Austrian immigrant could never hold office in America? Or where would our country be if all the space exploration experts listened when all those other experts said you can't put a man on the moon?

So, when you come to me at Providence Fit Body Boot Camp and you do the program, and I map out your nutrition plan, and if you tell me you can't follow the plan or do a push up, I dismiss the statement with a "you can and you will" response. I am regularly reminding people that if one human being is capable of performing a certain task, almost all of us are, and you need to change the negative mindset in order to achieve your goals, whether in fitness or life in general.

What makes one human being more successful or healthier, or more educated, or more fit than another? It's usually because the fit guy never said, "I can't work out because of my busy schedule" or the successful one never said, "I can't make it happen," or the educated one never thought "I can't pass this class."

How it starts

When you throw your hands in the air and say, "I can't," you won't, because many things require mental positivity equal to physical strength. Many exercises require mental focus to make the mind-muscle connection, which in turn promotes body awareness, creating better balance and muscle control. So when you enter with a negative mindset you will fail, because by saying you can't, you have given up hope, and refusing to try eliminates all chances for success.

I must have said this to someone recently in my boot camp because I overheard a client say, "I don't think I can do this, but I can't tell Matt because he'll get mad, so I am going to try." She said it jokingly, but tried to master the move because I motivated her to make an attempt. I told her in the beginning that the words "I can't" aren't allowed at my Fit Body Boot Camp, and now she is working harder, and I am confident she will see amazing results that wouldn't be possible if she had maintained the negative mindset. Remember this quote as you work forward toward your goal: *"You will miss 100 percent of the shots you don't take."*

29

IT'S ALL IN YOUR HEAD

Physically, I believe we are one of the most inferior species alive. Our skin is easily penetrable, we can't adapt to our surroundings when seasons change, our throats and heads are exposed to danger, and we can't really protect ourselves without some sort of weaponry. Think about living in the wild — fighting a lion, or wild boar with your bare hands, or wrestling a gorilla — see what I mean? Our survival as a species has been due to the evolution of our brains — our intelligence. Adaptation hasn't happened in the way it usually does for most species. We don't grow thicker fur in the winter, nor do we shed it in the summer. We don't hibernate for an entire season (though with these winters lately, it seems like a good idea). We survive because we are able to create ways to survive in our element. We build shelters, often using up valuable natural resources to do so. At one time, and still today, we depend on the use of toxic elements to provide heat. We clothe ourselves with a lot of synthetic material made with toxic dyes to keep us warm. You don't see animals putting on sweaters and gloves, or hiding in heated shelters to escape the cold, but we need to. We can't fly south, either — at least not with our own natural abilities. So instead, we figured out how to fly using giant flying machines that also use mass amounts of toxic fuel, and leave toxic emissions in our atmosphere, all in our quest to escape colder climates.

Adaptation & Extinction

Once again, our intelligence and abilities have created ways for us to survive as a species. So why are we sicker, heavier, less athletic, and overall becoming less healthy? Our intelligence levels seem to be diminishing over time, because we do know better, yet we continue to find ways to push ourselves into extinction. Let me elaborate.

A few years ago, the state of California put out a bill that would require food companies to list the fact that GMOs were present in their products. That got shot down. Instead, food companies that do not use GMOs have to label their products GMO free, so we can avoid the unhealthy ingredients in our food supply. While I'm not a scientist, I spend a lot of time looking at the types of food we eat — and I don't look at the front of the package — I look at the back. I read ingredients. And I look for food source information. GMOs, in my opinion, are polluting our food supply chain. And what's more, once the origins of our food — the seed — gets modified, there is literally no going back. If we, as a species, have evolved our brains to know how to survive, then we should know that we don't want to eat food modified or made in a lab with artificial, or genetically modified ingredients. Again, I ask, if we are so smart, why didn't this bill pass? Why aren't we aggressively going after a natural food supply chain? Instead, we are allowing food manufacturers to continue to put additives and chemicals in our food, and manipulate the industry. We allow them to manipulate our minds and our buying behaviors, too.

Remember the proposed ban in New York City on the Big Gulp soda? The big guns — the food companies — came out and convinced us that somehow our rights were being violated, and the ban never happened. We are facing close to a 35 percent obesity rate in this country, and the consumption of soda and sugary foods are the main reason why. We've focused so much on fat — saturated, trans, mono, and good/bad fats — that we have overlooked the supreme violator in our diets — sugar.

How smart are you?

But we are supposed to be the most intelligent species, right? Yet, we're watching our food supply be contaminated by natural substances such as sugar or by pesticides and even genetically altering the makeup of the origins of our foods. We're not listening to the great minds we spend so much educating. We're not listening to what is even greater — our instinct. Eating natural foods is safer. Avoiding medication when you can do things, naturally, to be well, is better. The concept of taking a pill to lower our cholesterol, or meds to maintain our sugar levels and fight diabetes, is one that has become mainstream — and we know that the majority of our greatest diseases are lifestyle controllable and preventable. Yet, we don't listen to our great minds enough. We avoid listening to our instinctual voices. We are caught up in the easy fix to our problems. And, in trying to make life easier, we have made it harder and more troubling to our planet and future generations.

I don't know what is happening, or why. We as humans are an inferior species on many levels, but our intelligence has allowed us to survive, and thrive. Are we going backwards? — cloning fish, manufacturing food, eating stuff we know will make us sick. We take pills that disclose the harmful side effects as they are shouted at us over the pretty television commercials of people sitting in bathtubs looking at sunsets. We're doing irreparable harm to our soils and oceans. Companies are in a war fighting advocates that try to keep us safe and healthy. With the internet, and all the information out there, ignorance is no longer an excuse. In the end, it is an individual decision each of us must make for ourselves and our family. Laws and regulations will only do so much. So I ask you, if you are so smart, why aren't you healthy? And what are you going to do about it — today?

30

IT'S JUST TALK...

In my business, I hear sayings and clichés all the time, and when you surf through social media, especially marketing sites that want to sell you fitness stuff, you see many. Most of the time when I hear people talking about these unproven bits of advice, their friends are usually nodding in agreement with them — as if they are the owners of some meaningful philosophy. I like to take things literally, so I am going to shoot some holes in two of these bits of "advice," share my take on the subject matter, and give you something to think about.

1. "Getting to the gym is half the battle"

NO, it's not! Most people will tend to agree with this, without giving it much thought, but I am here to tell you that just getting to the gym isn't even close to winning half the battle. As a matter of fact, just showing up isn't even 10 percent of the battle. I have been watching people "show up" at gyms for over 20 years and get nowhere close to their goals due to their lack of drive, discipline, and direction. When you go to the gym it takes knowledge, programming, and hard work, with plenty of strenuous exercise and sweat to see any results at all. After you establish what it takes, it requires consistency to even get close to winning the battle. Just think about it — would you say, "just showing up at the market, is half the battle to eating healthy?" When in reality, you can go very wrong if you do not have a list, or a plan, or an idea about what is good for you and what is not. So if you think that just showing up at a gym, sitting on a lifecycle, lumbering around the free weight floor, or reading a magazine on a treadmill is going to help you gain ground with your battle, you are sadly mistaken. At my Fit Body Boot Camp, or anywhere where you are working with a qualified professional, you aren't going to gain much ground with an attitude like that. There should be a plan for you when you walk in the door. At my gym, I give you direction, hold you accountable, and provide all the tools you need to conquer your challenges and achieve results. No, it's not good enough to just show up. Be prepared. For what? To sweat, and move, and work hard, because overcoming poor conditioning requires a lot more than just showing up.

2. "Great abs are made in the kitchen"

OK so there is some merit to this quote, but just eating great isn't going to put muscle on your body and make you fit. Lifting weights and bouts of high intensity training will. I know a few people who eat correctly, but their bodies are still mush. Abdominals are a muscle group and need to be trained to get stronger and look better, just like back and biceps. Besides, you can over eat quality food just as easily as overeating junk food. Granted you will be healthier, but it is impossible to get fit without exercise. You need to burn body fat and build muscle to achieve your fitness goals, and you can't do it with good nutrition alone. You need to shed some sweat, move some weight, and feel the burn to complete the package. Yes, the phrase, "you can't out exercise a bad diet" is true, but "you can't eat your way to total fitness" is also true.

I am not trying to discourage anyone, but I am trying to give you a reality of the whole concept of fitness. I never sugar coat (pun intended) things so I am telling you that being fit and maintaining your health is hard work, and no easy task, regardless of what all the clichés on the street are telling you.

31

IT'S NOT EASY

B eing fit and healthy isn't easy. There are many personal obstacles as well as outside distractions that derail us from our
mission, and I am here to help you overcome them. It is difficult enough for people who *like* to work out to find the time, and
for people who want to eat healthy, who also have to eat on the go,
to do so. Tough it is for the uninformed and unmotivated.

Obstacle #1 — marketing and advertising

Everyone wants to get results the quickest way possible and do the
least amount of work. And I have said it over and over again that
there is no easy way. It takes time, energy, and intensity to be fit.
You will not get it in four minutes a day, or by eating some sandwich with Fritos in it because some guy claims he lost 100 pounds
eating at a fast-food chain. You won't get abs in eight minutes a day
without a proper eating plan, and you will not get fit at home
watching videos unless you follow the program with intensity and
read the fine print. So, do not give in to all the fancy ads — if it says
easy or quick, it is a lie. It is hard work, but anything worth having
is worth hard work. Many people fall prey to these quick fix
schemes, and when they fall short of unrealistic goals, they become
discouraged and quit. So do not start a program with unrealistic
goals, and remember, there is really no easy way.

Obstacle #2 — peer pressure

People who are jealous of your aesthetics find fault and make fun of what you are doing. They harass you when you order healthy food, or read a label, or make a comment about working out. You get the "Not everyone can look like you" statement in condescending overtones, and they roll their eyes when someone compliments you. There are reasons why you are fit, and they are not because you are busier or have more important things than they do going on in their lives. Fitness people all have a naysayer, and I say ignore the negativity and let them rant, because it makes as much sense as mocking someone with more money than you. Take jealousy as a compliment, and stick to your game plan. Being fit and healthy is nothing to be ashamed of or embarrassed about, and it is a lifestyle you shouldn't have to justify or defend. When I hear that I am too fitness conscious or that I let fitness run my life, or that I take it too far, I don't feel the need to explain myself, nor do I have the desire to critique negative aspects of someone else's lifestyle. I feel that taking care of yourself is a normal, primal instinct, and feel that knowingly consuming products that are harmful or damaging to your body is not in your best interest, so know that you are doing the right thing, stay the course, and let your critics enjoy their doctors' visits.

Obstacle #3 — eating on the go

Eating on the go seems to be the toughest challenge for both healthy individuals and foodies. It isn't impossible to do, but it does take a conscious effort and a little planning. It can be done. So don't make excuses like lack of time or restaurant meetings be an excuse to do it wrong. My first suggestion is to find a good market. Most have eating areas and prepared food ready and available. A roasted chicken and a salad or vegetables makes a perfect lunch and usually leaves extra for later. This costs about the same as a sandwich and bag of chips and is healthier and more balanced. There are several types of Tex/Mex chains that offer a decent meal on the go. I suggest getting bowl type meals with beans, instead of the wrap, and pile on the veggies. Many ethnic spots offer the same type of fare with meals being available as an alternative to the standard sandwich or greasy processed meal. Although this isn't as good as buying organic food and making it yourself, it is an acceptable alternative.

There are many ways to be deterred from a healthy lifestyle. We live in a time of what's becoming the worst man-made health epidemic ever. Disease and obesity are on the rise and our food supply keeps getting worse, but I do not write to discourage people — only to motivate and educate. I try to give you the tools to make the right choices and make positive gains. It's up to you to open the toolbox.

32

IT'S NOT YOUR FAULT...

If you know me and how I operate, you know that I have very little tolerance for excuses or b.s. stories. I truly believe that if you want something, or want to do something badly enough, you CAN find a way. If you do not want it badly enough, you will make up an excuse. And every excuse has an anecdote. "I didn't have time to hit the gym," is a common one. I counter that with, "You had the same 24 hours that everyone else did, you just decided to spend yours differently, and did not schedule 45 minutes of your day to workout. But you HAD the time." Another that folks like to use is, "I can't afford to eat healthy, or join a gym." My answer, "If you have an iPhone, cable TV, eat out, buy coffee daily from a coffee shop, drink any amount of alcohol regularly, or own sneakers that cost $100 or more, then you CAN afford it... but you choose not to include health and taking care of yourself into your budget." Yes, organic food costs more, but when you are trying to improve your physique, and overall health, you won't be buying all the costly, processed junk food anymore either, so it balances out. Again, if you want something bad enough, you can find a way to make it happen.

However, there is one excuse you can get away with for not reaching your fitness and fat loss goals — and that is ignorance. If you truly don't know about something, or you were misled into believing something was healthy, or you were lured into some heavily marketed gimmick, I'll give you a pass, because the world is full of trickery and false claims. I tell all my clients that you can only use this excuse once with me, because when you become a member of my Fit Body Boot Camp, I not only provide you with kick-ass, stimulating, and fun workouts, I try to educate you and explain step by step how to reach all your health and fitness goals. During every member's nutrition consultation, I explain all the benefits and pitfalls of different foods, and how they react inside your bodies, how they affect your blood glucose/sugar, and what types/brands of foods are good and bad. We also talk about how to accelerate your metabolism by eating frequently, and how to balance nutrients. When you leave our consultation, you will have a better understanding about what makes us fit versus what makes us fat. Then the "I didn't know" statement becomes obsolete, because now you know, and if you still continue down the path of destruction, well, that WILL BE your fault.

One of the biggest misunderstandings I hear frequently is, "but I shop at Whole Foods so I eat healthy." First, I want to say that I shop there, and only there. I enjoy shopping at Whole Foods because you CAN find all sorts of healthy, quality food that you can't find anywhere else, BUT everything in the store isn't healthy or Fit Body approved. Just because a package of cookies is "organic" doesn't make it healthy, and it certainly won't help you when trying to get fit. It just means that the ingredients are better than the cookies that large food factories produce, and chemicals or GMOs aren't being used in their products. Better, yes, but not good. If you buy their conventional produce not labeled "organic," you may still be exposed to pesticides, and chemicals. The same goes for their animal products. You still need to pay attention and only purchase items with an animal welfare rating of four or better. Not all items in the store are the same quality, so you can't shop blind just because you are in a higher quality market. They also sell lots of beverages loaded with sugar and calories, and this is a big no-no in my book. Unless it's a smoothie packed with (measured) healthy nutrients, and protein, I do not recommend drinking anything containing calories. Even organic soda, and sports drinks. When you drink calories, they usually find their way to your hips, belly, and butt. And fast! It is very easy to pack on extra pounds just by consuming one calorie packed beverage a day, even if the label says it is good for you. Don't fall into the liquid calorie trap and eat your calories. Drinking excess calories is too easy.

I got the idea for this column yesterday when I was at Whole Foods eating lunch. I overheard a couple of women talking about how hard they are trying to lose weight, and how they are eating salads as part of their effort. When I got up, I had to look at what they were eating, and to my disappointment, I saw two huge salads, topped with approximately 1500 calories worth of cheese, beans, olives, eggs, beets, seeds, and nuts, along with some sort of dressing covering the whole thing. It was a real struggle not to say something, but I learned a long time ago not to offer my advice unless asked or retained to do so. Number one, I don't want to look like a know it all, and number two, I didn't want to discourage two strangers making what they thought was a valiant effort to lose weight. It was obvious that they wanted to better themselves but didn't know how. This is the case with a lot of folks. They try but fail due to lack of knowledge. This is the only excuse for not being able to achieve perfect health and fitness. But once you come into my facility, remember, you are only allowed to use this excuse once. I will help you learn. My advice? Before you exert any effort in anything you do, do some research or hire a trained professional. Let someone help you reach whatever goal you have as efficiently and effectively as possible. Time is too valuable to waste, so stop going around in circles, and follow the straight line to success.

33

JOIN THE RESISTANCE!

J oin the resistance is a term or mantra used by one of my favorite motivators, Martin Rooney, founder of the Training for Warriors program. He is a guy who created a system of training for MMA fighters and athletes. He now uses his knowledge and enthusiasm to teach personal trainers to be better at what they do. I have attended many of his seminars, as well as completed his certification program, and although his technical knowledge about training and nutrition isn't more advanced than mine, he has still made me a better trainer by transferring energy, passion, and motivation to my skill set. We both believe in the work hard/smart, eat and rest well theory, and use the same common-sense approach.

So, what does he mean by "join the resistance?" Is he preparing us for a live version of the terminator, or some anti-government movement? No — the resistance is us (trainers and educators) trying to bring out the best in people and inspire them to be the best they can be. We motivate people to get up and exercise, eat quality food, get plenty of rest, take responsibility for their actions, and make changes for the best, both physically and mentally. To do this you have to resist laziness, temptation, and negative thought processes. I joined his resistance long ago, and now I am here to tell you how to fight the resistance.

Be strong against those working against you

As a personal trainer I encounter negative, overweight and/out of shape people who consider me and those who live this profession, neurotic, over board, too strict, and who take health and fitness too far — just because we take care of ourselves and live out our passion. This is the resistance we need to fight — the negatives — the thoughts and actions that work against us. When I am out socially, or with family, and someone says, "Eat this dessert" (usually some chemical laden fake food from a supermarket chain), "you need to live a little," it drives me crazy. I go out of my way and encourage others to have the knowledge and discipline to avoid these foods — so, how is this living it up? Eating something that is going to make me tired, feel lousy, maybe feed disease and sabotage the time I spent working out is not living it up in my book. But! Eating a nice medium rare filet, or getting a good night's sleep, IS! So, join me — and let's fight the resistance.

Choose the lesser evil

I was with my nephew at a Cub Scout campfire, and he wanted to eat a burnt marshmallow on a graham cracker with chocolate. I couldn't let him eat a carcinogenic piece of high fructose corn syrup on a stick just because all the other campers and parents were cooking them up and eating them. So I strategically dropped it in the fire and let him eat the cracker and chocolate. The lesser evil! Just because everyone does it, doesn't make it OK — Fight the Resistance!

It's your choice

When you are out with friends, and you stay out later than you wanted to, or you drank too much maybe due to peer pressure, or you get the" c'mon let's have one more," or "I don't like to drink alone, or just one shot for old times," remember — you are the one who has to suffer the next day. You will be dehydrated, tired, have a headache, and feel nauseous — you will be useless and miserable

because you didn't show enough discipline. It's your choice —
Fight the Resistance.

Fight for what you think is right

So for some populations joining the resistance means taking a stand
and fighting FOR what you think is right, and trying to instill methods of accountability, discipline, and self-worth into people, and to
shed a light on healthy living as a good thing that you can attain,
enjoy, and feel good about. For others, fighting the resistance
should mean avoiding something bad because everyone else is doing it — not giving in to peer, or society pressure, and making the
right choices. It's all about you doing it for yourself, because no one
else is going to do it for you. Big business food manufacturers don't
want you to eat healthy food because there is no profit in it for
them. Even healthcare settings are said to be more about managing
illness than keeping you healthy. It's the same with big pharma.
Imagine what could happen to specialties like orthopedic surgery
if we all trained well and learned how to move properly and avoid
injury? If everyone eats healthy, exercises properly, and gets plenty
of rest, much of this will be needed.

It's your war

It's time to fight the resistance. It's your war, and you need to fight
it. If you are following me on social media, or on my blog, you are
probably one of the 14 percent of people who work out. That's
right, only 14 percent of this country's population work out, so
we (people who care about our health) are the minority. I say if
you are a trainer or health professional, join the resistance. All
others? Fight the resistance.

34

LIFE IS NOT
A DRESS REHEARSAL...

I recently read a letter Steve Jobs wrote and I am sharing it with you. I think it is timely and significant enough because it directly relates to my life's mission. That mission is to help as many people as possible become as fit and healthy as they possibly can, and achieve great personal success doing it. Steve Jobs achieved massive success, but beyond creating a superior product, how many lives did he impact, personally, along the way? How many of his customers and coworkers did he see smile and get excited as a direct result of the positive influence he had on their lives? Yes, of course, buying tech toys makes us happy, but you know what I'm getting at. How did he enhance people's self-esteem, or make them feel physically invigorated? He may have given lots of money to useful causes, but did he have a deeper involvement to see the end result — how his support impacted people? I know I do, and money can't buy that type of satisfaction, the type that comes from knowing you made a difference in others' lives.

We get one chance; no retakes

I took his message personally, and I think you should too. He had little joy in his life despite all his wealth and success, because he had no balance; it was all work and chasing success. Yes, I want success, but I don't want to be miserable, and stressed out of my mind along the way. Health is invaluable, and Jobs regretted not taking better care of himself. This is why I wanted to share this with you. Don't reach that point in your quest for success, because once you are sick to a certain degree, it's highly unlikely you will bounce back. If you are overweight, sedentary, and live a destructive life-style, it is almost inevitable that you will travel along that path. Re-alize that being proactive and taking care of yourself now is the thing to do, instead of being reactive and trying to fix things when it's too late. So here it is. Grab a box of tissue, and read Steve Jobs' last words. Chase success, work hard, but create some balance while you are doing it. Do it for your kids, spouse, family, and more importantly, create that balance for — yourself! Unlike a movie, life has no dress rehearsal, cuts, or retakes. We only get one chance at this performance, so put your best foot forward, and cherish what's important to you.

Steve Jobs' Last Words

"I reached the pinnacle of success in the business world. In others' eyes, my life is an epitome of success. However, aside from work, I have little joy. In the end, wealth is only a fact of life that I am accustomed to. At this moment, lying on the sick bed and recalling my whole life, I realize that all the recognition and wealth that I took so much pride in, have paled and become meaningless in the face of impending death. In the darkness, I look at the green lights from the life supporting machines and hear the hum-ming mechanical sounds, I can feel the breath of God, of death, drawing closer... Now I know, when we have accumulated sufficient wealth to last our lifetime, we should pursue other matters that are unrelated to wealth... Should be something that is more important: Perhaps relation-ships, perhaps art, perhaps a dream from younger days... Non-stop pur-suing of wealth will only turn a person into a twisted being, just like me. God gave us the senses to let us feel the love in everyone's heart, not the illusions brought about by wealth. The wealth I have won in my life I can-not bring with me. What I can bring is only the memories precipitated by love. That's the true riches which will follow you, accompany you, giving you strength and light to go on. Love can travel a thousand miles. Life has

no limit. Go where you want to go. Reach the height you want to reach. It is all in your heart and in your hands. What is the most expensive bed in the world? — 'The Sick Bed'... You can employ someone to drive the car for you, make money for you, but you cannot have someone to bear the sickness for you. Material things lost can be found. But there is one thing that can never be found when it is lost — 'Life'. When a person goes into the operating room, he will realize that there is one book that he has yet to finish reading — 'The Book of Healthy Life'. Whichever stage in life we are at right now, with time, we will face the day when the curtain comes down. Treasure love — for your family, love for your spouse, love for your friends... Treat yourself well. Cherish others."

35

LIVING ON EASY STREET?

"I'm too tired, I don't have time, I don't like to work out, I'm too busy, I have kids, I know I need to but..." Excuses! These are some of the excuses people give for their excessive weight or poor health, for not working out, and for the lack of motivation and discipline it takes to get fit and healthy. My philosophy is and always has been, that if other people can find the time and do it, so can you. Stop justifying something you know is wrong, and work on self-improvement — now!

Excuses, Excuses, Excuses...

Don't wait until next Monday... OR for your kids to get older... OR for the New Year... OR *forget it*! I'm not buying it and no one else is either. Buck up and make a start now. I remember hearing a presenter at a workshop say that doing things that give instant gratification such as eating tasty junk food, hitting the snooze button, and pouring that second drink, are the things that are going to ruin your attempt at doing something good for yourself. It's often the tension and anticipation you experience by inaction that is the most stressful. Once you begin something, it gets to be part of your routine and you will achieve positive results. All that angst you put yourself through won't be there anymore — it will be replaced by a sense of control over your life. Once you change your mindset, and start to recognize that you can do something as long as you lose the excuses, self-improvement becomes attainable. A little positive mindset, guidance, hard work, and discipline will go a long way, and within a few months, your path to health and fitness will not be a dream, it will be right there right in front of you.

Really think you can get great Abs in 7 Minutes?

Why aren't more people fit and healthy if that's all it takes? Today's society is used to taking the easy way out. Planning your meals and getting your sweat on is a chore and requires planning and discipline. Sitting around and eating from a drive thru does not. Marketing gimmicks thrive on this attitude, always offering something quicker and faster. "7 Minute Abs" is a perfect example of how people are brainwashed into thinking that if you do something for a few minutes a day, you will achieve positive results. Steve Jobs said, "If you look deeper into people you thought were overnight successes, you will realize that it didn't really happen overnight." The same goes for all those great-bodied spokespeople for products. They didn't sculpt them overnight.

The defeatist mindset and the "I can't" attitude have to go. Think about it a little more. If another human being can do it, so can you. Nothing is impossible if you put your mind into doing something. If you are not good at something, make it a goal to get good at it. I feel as though I am a great trainer, but not so good at technology and business, but I knew if I wanted to become more successful in life I need to get better at both. So, I took the chance and opened a Fit Body Boot Camp and training facility. I looked at other people doing it, and figured if they are doing it, so can I. If I tossed my hands in the air and said, "I can't," it would never have happened. I hear it all the time from successful people that if you wait around for the perfect time, you will be waiting a long time if not forever.

What's the perfect time?

I know it gets intimidating and scary at times, but there are ways around that. Hire a coach or find someone to do it with you. At my facility, you will have both. I'm here, personally, as your coach, and there's a roomful of people around me with the same intentions. With my franchise, I get the same kind of help. There are coaches I can talk to, and getting together with others where everyone has the same goal of helping people get fit and healthy and creating a successful business. Everyone has the ability. First realize the problem then take action. Do not wait for that perfect time because YOU KNOW it will never come. The perfect time is now — today — this minute. What will you do with it? Live and make yourself better today. Remember — no excuses!

36

MAKING SACRIFICES

For our children

We have all done it at one time or another. We sometimes do it on a daily basis. Every good person makes sacrifices. If you have children, your life is a sacrifice. You have to sacrifice most of your time, money, and energy so you can take care of and insure that your child lives a happy, healthy, and productive life. Everything in your child's life depends on you and the amount of energy you put into their upbringing. If you do not make sacrifices, a problem child will arise and a lifetime of heartbreak could follow.

For our family

If you have elderly parents, or someone in your family gets sick, you will be making many sacrifices in your life to help them unless you are fortunate enough to afford full-time help. You may even live in a certain place that you don't like just to be close to your family, or you may forgo a well needed vacation just to attend a friend's wedding or an event for a child in the family. These are all examples of the sacrifices we make to please others; those instances when we put someone's needs or happiness before our own.

But — what about YOU?

But the one sacrifice you should not make and be completely selfish about is maintaining good health, and taking care of YOU. This doesn't mean that you will eat quality food and your family eats junk or that you deprive anyone of the essentials. This means that when it comes to your health, you should be #1. You can't take care of others unless you can first take care of yourself. It's like they tell you on an airplane, "Put on YOUR oxygen mask first before you assist someone else." I like this analogy because it correlates well to your own health and fitness, meaning that if you are sick or have ailments yourself, you can't be too helpful to others.

When I hear my friends say, "I do not have time to exercise because all my time is devoted to my kids," I ask them how much time their kids will spend with them if they have a heart attack and die? Or how useful are you if you are too heavy to play ball or go swim with them? That usually opens their eyes, and gets them thinking. Besides setting a good example, living healthy makes you a happier and more productive person, and that will make everyone better off. Eating healthy shouldn't be unattainable or too expensive. If you and your spouse are living well, driving new cars, going out for dinner frequently, and your kids belong to every sport and activity available, then think about your priorities. If expense is your reason for letting your health diminish, you need to reassess the situation. Make cuts to your time and budgets accordingly so you can eat right and exercise.

Sacrificing your health for others is the wrong sacrifice to make. Your health and well-being should be your main priority in life over family, money, work and friends. It is OK to put yourself first in this one particular instance because it will translate to a better you, and this will give off positive energy. And you will be teaching your family lifelong habits that will benefit them, too. If people see your dedication as a little selfish, then let them know that it is more selfish if you don't put your health first because you will eventually burden others with your own ailments, and require others to sacrifice for you.

As with most things, lead by example. It will mean less sacrifice for everyone in the long run.

37

Yes,
The Planet's in Trouble
But So Are We.

Today, I am writing this article not thinking as a personal trainer but thinking as a scientist from Mars. I'm looking down on Earth and the people who live there, studying their behaviors, before we decide whether we want to inhabit Earth or destroy it. This study is being conducted to examine the habits, strengths, and weaknesses of the human population so we can make an informed decision if this is what we want for our people. We will observe these beings from different parts of the Earth and discuss their lifestyles.

We zero in on the United States, and the first thing we notice is that they use noisy devices to purposely disrupt their circadian cycles and deprive themselves of necessary sleep. Then they jump up without stretching muscles that were tightened by lack of blood flow to a body that was in a relaxed supine position. They don't drink enough water, and after several hours, they become dehydrated. Even their little hairy pets have enough common sense to stretch and hydrate after a long duration of inactivity. We watch as a large majority of these humans get dressed and put these tight uncomfortable objects on their feet, eat some sort of processed matter, drink an acidic beverage, and rush out the door, sleep deprived and malnourished.

Most drive themselves and their children to a place and congregate with others inside a sunlit-proof building surrounded by electromagnetic radio waves, purposely putting themselves in an environment that stresses them out and makes them unhappy. They then perform tasks for an eight-hour span of time, only stopping to eat more man-made processed snacks and substances. After they complete their eight hours, some go back home and sit in front of another electronic device, and others go to a place, also lacking natural sunlight, full of weighted machines to perform mundane tasks such as walking or rowing in place over and over again for specific periods of time. They're not going anywhere, and they're putting their bodies at risk by pushing heavy weights around aimlessly, again and again. How curious.

When that's all done, they feed their bodies more unbeneficial substances, and some are now drinking, but instead of water, they consume alcoholic beverages that cause havoc to all the systems in the human body. After another session on another electronic device, these humans will consume some sweet addictive substance then attempt to fall asleep. After hours of failure, some grab on to curious pills to help them sleep, or that will help them wake up in the morning. They are in a vicious cycle of causing themselves harm. This cycle continues daily, until sickness or death occurs.

In conclusion, based on the observational data collected, we have determined that despite all the knowledge these humans have access to, that due to lack of discipline, addiction, availability of, and amount of harmful food produced, we have decided that this harmful way of life is not appealing enough for us to want to live among them. And rather than waste our ammunition to destroy Earth, our data indicates that humans will eventually all just destroy themselves. We will move on.

I wish there was a blockbuster movie made like this. Sadly, this is how our life would appear — though it's considered a normal way of life for a lot of people. Just changing your eating habits and improving exercise efficiency can greatly improve your quality of life and have you feeling better in as little as two weeks. This doesn't have to be difficult; the information is out there. Call a pro or do your own research — you'll be glad you did. With all the emphasis on global warming and pollution and the saving of our planet, are WE — each of us — not due a check-up of our own vessels, our bodies, and a whole new way of living healthy?

38

NO TIME.
TOO BUSY.
FAIL.

I t starts with motivation. Then it's all about time management. You *can* improve your health in just 90 minutes every day.

"I just don't have the time to hit the gym. I am too busy to pre-pare my meals for the day." When I hear people say these things, it is usually the beginning of a debate. I will ask the question, "what is more important than your health?" And the answer is: "You just don't understand what it's like to have my schedule." So I usually reply with something like: "If you want it bad enough you will find a way, and if you don't, you will find an excuse." I also tell this person that if they are serious and want to make a little effort with their time management, and supply some discipline and motiva-tion, I can and will help them achieve their goals. Here are some examples of how you can jumpstart your path to health and fitness with just diet changes.

Failing to prepare is preparing to fail

Preparation is the key to time management when you have a busy schedule, so that's why we need do certain tasks ahead of time. It all starts with the grocery store or market. Go in knowing exactly what you will be consuming throughout your day. Make a list beforehand and give some real thought to it. When you enter the store, you'll have a plan to go right to it. Do not let yourself wander and aimlessly shop, because that's a great way to buy foods you do not need, waste a bunch of time, and spend more money. Now that you have all the nutritious food you need, it's time to prepare for consumption.

Cook it up

Ever notice how efficiently restaurants operate? They prepare food in an assembly line or keep food cut up in a hold unit. So to be efficient, we should do the same. When you unpack your groceries, leave stuff like carrots and strawberries on the counter, then go wash and prep a few days' worth before you put them away. Cut up some kale, and have it ready to cook. Hard boil a few eggs for some ready to eat muscle-building protein. If you look at my daily Facebook postings (Matt Espeut or Providence Fit Body Boot Camp) you'll see lots of eggs. I don't make them each and every time I have breakfast, lunch or dinner, I make them ahead of time so the cooking process doesn't get in the way of my nutrition plan. You can also weigh and portion your meats so you know exactly how much you are eating. You can prep a couple of days' worth of snacks and meals in about 30 minutes. There is no excuse not to.

Work it out

I believe exercise is important but your nutrition is more important. That is the first thing you need to focus on to achieve your goals, but you still need some movement to maintain function and fitness. Even if you do not have time to go to the gym, you should do some sort of activity to ramp up your heart rate and get your body moving. You could piece together six or seven body weight moves and perform 15-minute workouts by moving in a circuit, nonstop, for the entire time. This will help you build some muscle, burn fat and feel great about yourself — all for a 15-minute investment. Another excuse gone... out the window!

What will you do in the next 90 minutes?

Folks, being fit and healthy is only a few simple lifestyle modifications away. I just gave you a few examples of how to improve your fit levels in less than 90 minutes' time. There are 1440 minutes total in a day. You should be able to invest less than 10 percent of them to become leaner and stronger. If not, then you don't want it bad enough and you will find an excuse. If that's the case, then focus on motivating yourself. Find some old pictures of a fit and trim and healthy you. Look at your children or your spouse. Use vanity and buy something to wear that you love but right now doesn't look good on you and hang it up where you can see it every day. Believe it or not, those wannabe photos on the fridge work. Assuming you are motivated, find 10 percent of the hours of this day, and as Nike says, "Just do it!"

39

ONE STEP AT A TIME

I t's the small things that make a big difference in both positive and negative ways. We all know that trying to live a healthy lifestyle is a big commitment. Overall, it seems like an unattainable goal for most. You need to be constantly buying fresh food, paying attention to everything you eat, finding time to exercise, and when you do find time, taking a lot of effort to make it through a workout.

The same goes when trying to be successful in your career. It's a big task. Long hours and schedules full of work. When you look at the whole picture, these are huge mountains to climb, but you can't get to the top in one giant step. It takes lots of smaller steps to get to there.

One of the first steps you need to take is to start eliminating small negatives that effect your health or life in general. One example — I was with my cousin the other day and she ordered an iced coffee with extra-extra cream and extra-extra sugar. She wants to lose some weight so I informed her that cutting four of these drinks weekly would reduce her empty calorie consumption by 1000. Another small change you could make would be to pack your own lunch. You would be able to eat quality food, measure the proper amount, and have an added plus by saving about $8 a day. And, you would save yourself some time by not spending half of your lunch break getting your food. Another small step in your quest for health could be to get to bed on time. The benefits of a good night's rest are invaluable and include increased energy, elevated mood, cellular repair, and muscle growth. This is a habit change that has no cost to it at all.

Eating breakfast is another small yet important habit. When we sleep, we basically fast, so to not have anything to eat before starting your day will not only lower your energy levels, it slows your metabolism causing you to store more and burn less body fat. This can be avoided by eating two hard-boiled eggs (prepare them the night before) and some fruit, and you have a quick healthy jump-start to your day. Another small step that is time efficient is to crank up a couple of short 15 to 30-minute workouts during the week. You could do a non-stop body weight / plyometric workout just about anywhere, and even if you already hit the gym, these workouts will torch body fat while maintaining muscle.

Yes, you *can*...

In doing what I do, I hear a lot of excuses and reasons why people "can't." I take it as part my job to make people believe that they "can." If you pile a mound in front of someone to climb, they will most likely fail. But if you present this mound one stone at a time, the intimidation factor diminishes and the success rate rises. I say conquer your fitness and health goals by seeing them as one small positive change at a time. But it's YOU who must initiate and take that first step. Once you do, there's help out there to keep going. Success takes time on all levels.

40

PREVENT THAT PLATEAU IN THE FIRST PLACE

I made a good analogy yesterday when I was talking to one of my clients about losing weight and reaching her goal. I told her that you can compare building yourself to building the perfect lawn. It's difficult in the beginning, but when you hit your goal, the maintenance gets easier.

She was on point with her food and exercise program, and lost over 20 pounds doing everything correctly and being precise with her nutrition plan. But, now she is at a standstill, and the weight loss has hit a plateau. This is not uncommon. After digging into the issue at hand, she confessed that she wasn't eating perfectly, but couldn't understand why the weight loss was not happening as rapidly.

So, I hit it home with her that every time she ate something bad or had too many calories that it would halt progress. It usually won't make you go backwards, but every bad decision you make while trying to achieve your goal is like hitting a speed bump in the road. Using the perfect lawn example, I said that in order to have a beautiful manicured lawn, you need to dig up the crab grass, kill the grubs, dig up and spread new loam, rake it, level it, plant seed, and water it relentlessly, until it's where you want it to be. After the initial hard work and labor, it's easier to maintain. All you need to do is water, fertilize, and cut it.

Reaching your weight loss goal is no different. It's a lot of hard work and discipline until you get there. You need to be religious-like with your eating and workout regularly. Building muscle and burning fat takes time, effort, desire, drive, and discipline. If you don't follow this format, it's like not watering that lawn on a hot day. It's going to halt progress or knock you back a step. You need to take a straight line, no-nonsense approach to reach your goal, or it takes longer to get there. Like I said earlier, the maintenance is easier, and here's why.

It takes time

Muscle takes time to develop. It takes you longer to build muscle than it does to burn fat. But once you develop muscle, it not only makes you look better and your clothes fit looser and hang in a more flattering way. But the biggest benefit is that it will elevate your metabolism. A pound of muscle is smaller in volume than a pound of fat, and it's metabolically a more active tissue so it will torch more calories at rest and make it easier to maintain your weight. But you still need to do the work to maintain your healthy and fit body.

It's not a part time job

Being fit is a lifestyle, not a part time job. You can't go all out "some-times," especially when you have a big goal to accomplish. You need to go even harder until you reach your goal. You can't coast to success, you need to get on the high-speed train and stay on it until you reach your destination. If you need to lose 40 pounds, and you get to the 20-pound point and then lose interest and slack off, you will plateau, or even worse, slowly regress. However, once you hit your goal, even if you slack off and put a pound or two back on during a vacation or holiday, you only have a short distance to go to get it back. My advice is when you need to reach your destination, go full speed ahead; once you get there, it's OK to go sightseeing. Make it happen first, then relax and enjoy it later.

Fitness is like a business

Success in fitness is a lot like success in business. I compare the two all the time because I am trying to be successful with both. I got the fitness down, and after 25 years in the industry, I can get you fit faster than anyone else, and I am very confident about that. Being in business is a different story. Although doing great 18 months out, I know I still have a lot to learn. Every month, my business does better, but I can't — and won't — coast just because I have a great month. I work relentlessly to reach my goals (even though my goal of success is undefinable). I am working just as hard as I did on day one, but I work differently now. I am building my team and growing to new levels, so I still work hard, but I work more efficiently. Once I reach a certain point, I won't coast, but the maintenance and flow of everyday operations will become more manageable and easier to organize, just like your perfect physique.

So, when you set a goal, go after it with everything you've got. Even when success shines a little, you can't rest and get complacent. We will always have temporary setbacks, but you need to make sure they stay that way — temporary. Always keep that positive "I can do mindset," and realize that anything is attainable if you work for it. Then when all the hard work is done, new habits will be created, and the maintenance will be as simple as brushing your teeth. It becomes part of your everyday life, and when you fall, getting up is a lot easier.

41

PROACTIVE. REACTIVE. YOUR CHOICE.

Today, I wanted to dig deeper and give you some more specific reasons why you need to start taking better care of yourself. I do a lot of preaching about the healthy lifestyle I can convert you to if you join my program and take my advice. It's not for vanity reasons, or just to lose weight, but to promote your overall health. Because you can look fit, lean, or thin and still be unhealthy (fitness competitors do it all the time), let's understand things correctly — first, health. Then, fitness.

Proactive/Reactive — and Diabetes

When you start paying closer attention to what a poor nutrition plan and a sedentary lifestyle will do to you, it will make you think about trying to be proactive and prevent things from going wrong, rather than being reactive and trying to fix things once you are broken.

Diabetes is one of the most common, preventable disease caused by poor nutrition and lifestyle. This disease wouldn't even exist if it weren't for sugar, processed food, and all the other garbage that big food companies are pushing into the marketplace. But it's too profitable for these companies and drug manufacturers to eliminate, so it's up to people like me to try and convince you that if you keep going down a destructive path, you will become a statistic. Read on

114

and hopefully you will see the light and make some positive changes in your life.

Type II Diabetes is the most common form of diabetes. There are 30.8 million children and adults in the United States, or 10 percent of the population, who have diabetes. While an estimated 19.6 million have been diagnosed with diabetes, unfortunately, only 11.2 million people (or nearly one-third) are unaware that they have the disease. In Type II Diabetes, either the body does not produce enough insulin or the cells ignore the insulin. Insulin is necessary for the body to be able to use sugar. Sugar is the basic fuel for the cells in the body, and insulin takes the sugar from the blood into the cells. When glucose (sugar) builds up in the blood instead of going into cells, it can cause problems. Right away, your cells may be starved for energy; over time, high blood glucose levels may hurt your eyes, kidneys, nerves or heart.

The Diabetic Scenario:

1. Calorie restriction, skipping meals, diet pills, and unbalanced meals consisting of mostly high glycemic carbohydrates
2. Stress response and altered hormonal levels
3. Immune response, digestive issues, increase insulin and cortisol response (two hormones that store fat around the midsection)
4. Elevated lipogenic (fat storing) enzymes and decreased lipolytic (fat burning) enzymes
5. Muscles become sensitive to insulin
6. Fat collection in the midsection, fatigue, Type II Diabetes and insulin resistance

Causes:

1. Eating a diet high in simple carbohydrates while low in fat and proteins
2. Eating a conventional diet of fast foods, boxed, canned or microwavable foods

3. Eating a diet high in sugar (either from candy or enriched breads / pastas)
4. A diet consisting of fruit juices (sugar water) or any form of soda
5. A diet that is low in water consumption
6. A sedentary lifestyle

Treatments:

1. Eliminate all boxed, canned, processed and microwavable foods
2. Eliminate all forms of sugars and high glycemic carbohydrates
3. Eat a diet of organic proteins and fats (fats slow down the insulin spike)
4. Get to bed by 10 p.m. and get up no earlier than 6 a.m.
5. Begin some form of exercise routine (boot camp, preferably)

If you are proactive in preventing diabetes in the first place, it is much easier to maintain a balanced state of health in the body. Fixing diabetes can be done. But it is hard and it takes much more effort than preventing it in the first place. The same goes for losing weight, getting your cholesterol down, and being fit. If you're fighting diabetes or other lifestyle disease, make a plan to fight your way back. If you are at high risk (diabetes in your family?) then be especially vigilant. If you're healthy now, then keep it that way.

See you in the gym.

42

REWARD YOURSELF

I *haven't had time to get to the gym. I haven't had time to call you back. I want to see that movie, but I don't have time. I want to start packing and bringing my lunch, but I don't have time. Haven't had time to stop over, but I will soon.*

Does this sound familiar to you? Heck, we can all relate to this. Right? Well, here are some other questions. If my gym always has people in it, and the phone is ringing throughout the day, I *do* usually have my food with me, and I *do* usually see my family members several days a week… it makes me wonder. After all, we are all given the same 24 hours in a day. So why do others have the time, or find the time, to do certain things? Why are other people working out regularly, almost no matter what else happens in their day? Why do some people almost always find the time to eat healthy food? Yes, I'll agree, it takes more time — time to think, plan, buy, cook, and sometimes pack. Why do some people get through their to-do list almost all the time, make all their phone calls that need to be made, and still get to enjoy a few of life's simple pleasures, like going to the movies, while others are always saying they just can't find the time?

MAKE the time

Why? Because people MAKE the time to do the things that are important or necessary to them. They do not get extra time during the day, nor do they have some magic wand that gets things done for them. They manage their time so they can be efficient and accomplish all the necessary things that are part of their day. If you want something bad enough, you will make the time to get it. If it isn't important enough, then you will just make an excuse. I know that there are certain things that we can't avoid such as kids getting sick and having to stay home from school — granted, you can't get out of the house. Your boss sets a deadline and you can't get out of it so you need to stay late, or you get into a car accident, and are stranded for a day with no vehicle. These are extraordinary circumstances, and can't be avoided; legitimate reasons to fall off track... temporarily. But, they are not part of our everyday routines and happen infrequently. Therefore we must deal with the temporary situation, fix the problem, and move on.

It's when you say, "I know I should be working out, but..." or "I know my diet isn't that good but..." or "I feel bad that I haven't seen this person in a while but..." These are the things you should be working to try and fix. Saying you do not have the time is a self-fabricated excuse because if others can find the time to do it, so can you. So why don't we do the things that are important to us? Why do we get discouraged when we don't get enough done in our day? When you fail to accomplish what you set out to do, day in and day out, it becomes a habit. We are all still doing things that we know are wrong. We say it to ourselves. We say it to friends. Heck, we even say it to strangers. My advice is to find one of those things that you know you are doing wrong, and stop doing it. Then, decide what is really important to you and make the time.

Time Management

Time is our most valuable asset, yet we seem to always be wasting it. There's a lot of information out there about how to be better at managing your time here are some tips that work for me — maybe they will work for you.

> 1. Make a list of everything you need to accomplish in any given day. I remember back to the days when I was a paperboy, my

supervisor would tell us, "Keep your book and you will always collect more money that way" and he was right. I always knew who owed what when it was written down. The same holds true for your eating. Write it down, and you will be surprised at the empty calories going onto that list.

2. Prioritize your list. Put your important items on top. This way you will accomplish these items first. Here's what's on my list today:

> ** market*
> ** drop off Jr. at practice*
> ** write my blog*
> ** gym*
> ** car wash*
> ** pick up Jr. from practice*

3. Delegate the things that someone else can do for minimal cost like housekeeping, landscaping, small odd jobs like painting, and washing the car. Use the time that you have to do the things only you can do, like making money, and taking care of your health.

4. Execute that list. Nothing feels better than checking-off things you have accomplished. An even better feeling is crumpling up a bunch of sticky notes that are complete.

So, next time someone asks you why you didn't do something, do not say, "I didn't have the time." Instead reply, "I mismanaged my day, and didn't make the time to do it. It wasn't important enough for me to get it done."

Now, get out and enjoy doing something you love to do. Because time is really all we have. Reward yourself!

43

First Things First
Setting Your Goal

There are many different programs and types of workouts in this continually evolving and confusing industry, and in order to get ideal results and avoid injury, you must select the system that works for you, by fitting your needs and abilities to your program. Your first question to yourself should be — WHY?

You need to determine your goals first, then you need to get the correct directions to reach these goals. Otherwise it is like getting into your car without a map or destination. You will end up wasting time energy and money, or even worse, end up with an unnecessary injury. You need to treat exercise as if you were taking medication. Too much is an overdose, and too little does nothing. You need the right amount for it to be effective. (Note, I never encourage medication, but this seems to illustrate the idea.)

So with that being said, I will try to correlate your potential goal with a method of training you can adopt.

Although everyone has different goals they want to achieve, three things are set in stone and apply to EVERYBODY.

1). You need a nutrition program based on whole organic foods and proper hydration.

2). You must strengthen the core, before loading the body.

3). You need to master basic movement patterns such as the squat, press, dead lift, and rotational moves.

These rules apply to everyone from the recreational exerciser to the highest endurance athlete. If you do not accomplish these three things first, you will be swimming against the current, and results will be tougher or non-existent.

What are your goals?

Examples of goals may go from wanting to be more fit with better posture, to being a better golfer or a football player, to entering a fitness contest or bodybuilding show — and winning. If you are content with your dimensions, and you just want to maintain strength and mobility, body weight exercises such as pull-ups, push-ups and body weight squats will do the trick. Add core routines like planks and bridges and you can create a routine and perform it anywhere. There are lots of progressions that can be added to create a more intense workout, or adding simple equipment such as bands and med balls to create even greater challenges.

Golf

I meet a lot of guys this time of year who tell me right away that they want to improve their golf game. Although you do not need to be athletic to play golf, having strong core stability, proper range of motion, spine mobility, and strong shoulder stabilizers are essential to avoiding injuries due to the sheer force needed to perform a strong drive. You need exercises that promote strength, flexibility, acceleration muscles as well as deceleration muscles to help stabilize the core under force. Strong legs are important but you need mobility and balance, so single leg exercises are helpful. Cable, rotary, and stability exercises will be beneficial to maintain range of motion and build power.

Other sports

Football, hockey, rugby or any other contact or lateral sport requires another level of intensity. If you don't have it and your opponent does, you have a problem. If you want to play hard, you need to train harder. Your off-season should consist of at least two power sessions containing heavy dead lifts, squats, and press variations, as well as two to three metabolic / core sessions. Agility ladders, jam balls, Plyo boxes, and push sleds are all beneficial tools to make athletes strong and metabolically fit. All these tools will only work if you bring intensity to every session. You can't get fit to the level you need for competitive sports if you don't have a never quit attitude and mental toughness. If you can't push yourself in the gym, and are unprepared at game time, you end up on the injury list. So, train hard and smart and you will play at a higher level.

Bodybuilding

Bodybuilders and fitness contestants need to forget life as they know it and devote their life to their body. This is the most calculated and measured form of training you can do. Food needs to be weighed, measured and portioned for every meal. Exercise needs to be scheduled and never missed. You need to pay attention, and understand how your body responds to certain foods, supplements and exercise. Your willpower around food has to be flawless. Giving up sugar, bread, and dairy completely, and following a regimented diet for 8 to 12 weeks is a mandatory commitment. This takes an extreme amount of discipline, and hard work, and sometimes requires high-risk practices such as dehydration and depletion to achieve certain aesthetics that will impress judges. Proceed with caution but a competition could be a good goal in and of itself. Even if you don't win or place, it will be a test of one's discipline that you can use to accomplish your other goals in life.

44

SET GOALS — NOT RESOLUTIONS

I haven't made a New Year's resolution and I won't. I can't. I can't because I spend every day trying to self-improve. What I do have are goals. I have a goal to be successful. I also have my own opinion as to what success is, and I take a step every day to get there. I put more pressure on myself and I do things that constantly push me out of my comfort zone because I know that once we get comfortable, we get complacent and then we stop pushing ourselves, and forward progress stops. I have a rough idea of where I want to be, and I have no control as to when it will happen.

Take responsibility

I feel that by making daily or weekly goals, and accomplishing them, puts us a day closer — and that's all I can control. Getting better doesn't have a deadline, nor is it a destination or a goal you can accomplish and be done with it. Rather, it's a mindset that goes on forever. Replace phrases like, "I'm trying" with, "I'm doing my best," or, "I can't," with, "I'm going to attempt it." Stop making excuses and don't blame others. Take responsibility for your actions.

I consider a New Year's resolution like a diet… temporary. We need to make life changes to be successful at whatever it is we do, like make more money, lose weight, or be a better coach or parent. We need to be constantly changing and evolving in order to get better. We need to always try to learn from others by observing the things that were successful and the things that failed. Making some loose promise just because it's the start of the new year is not only ridiculous, but unlikely to happen. We need to strive and work harder to get better every day. OK, it's fun to do and I always encourage people to make goals and set out to accomplish them, but they have more meaning and are more likely to happen when you set them on your own terms without outside pressure, or jump on some bandwagon because everyone is doing it.

Set goals

I usually set my fitness goals around my birthday, and tell myself that I will be in the best shape of my life by the time my birthday actually arrives — and on most years, it comes true with the exception of a few injuries I've had here and there. This method has been working for the past 10 years because I learn more and fix the mistakes I make every day. I am healthier now and leaner than when I was in my 30's. Most of the time people need the January 1st date to undo the downhill spiral they started at Thanksgiving. That's all it is! We do so much damage from then to the end of the year, that now, we aren't making a "New Year's" resolution, we are just fixing the damage caused by the holidays. The non-stop eating, drinking, staying up late, and stress sabotages everybody's fitness accomplishments in just a few weeks! I actually challenged my Fit Body Boot Camp clients to a zero-pound challenge for that period of time, just to try and prevent my people from losing their current results, and limit the amount of damage. Now the challenge for the next month is to undo the damage, then I will put them back on the "get a little better and stronger each workout" system I have developed. You see, even the new people that come in with a resolution will soon realize that they didn't sign up for a quick fix or a temporary solution, because it is my job to change their mindset by establishing realistic goals and lifestyle changes that will stay with them for the long haul.

Alright, then, everyone should have one resolution — and that is to try to get better every day… Period.

45

So, Tell Me How You Really Feel

How are you feeling? Feeling out of shape? Feeling tired and lazy all the time? Do your joints hurt? Are you irritable and grouchy all the time? Feeling depressed and have low self-esteem? Do you get out of breath just walking up the stairs or carrying groceries from your car to the house? Are you sick of how you look in clothes and in the mirror? Or even worse, do you have trouble fitting into your clothes? Do you run and hide when someone pulls out a camera? Are you dreading putting on a bathing suit? Do you get sick often? Has your sex drive diminished, or even worse, your spouse's? If you answered yes to any, most, or all of those questions, today is your lucky day because I have a solution for you.

Are you ready? Here it is, the solution to all your woes and ailments. It's the magic bullet, the too good to be true problem-solving way to better health and vitality. Sit down because here it comes... (Drum roll, please!)

STOP EATING GARBAGE — AND EXERCISE!

Yes, folks, exercise and good nutrition IS the answer to everything. It will make you feel better inside and out. It will give you more energy throughout your day, and when you have more energy, you become more productive. When you become more productive, you get more tasks done, and you become more efficient, and that can relate to being more organized, making more money, accomplishing your goals, and in the end, feeling better about yourself on all levels.

Diet

One of the key aliments people with poor eating habits experience is inflammation in the joints and in the digestive tract. One of the top selling drug categories is treatment for inflammation. Sure, you can take a pill, but be ready for side effects that will be worse than the symptoms they are treating. I listen to the commercials on TV, and when they roll off the disclaimer and the side effects at the end, I find myself yelling out loud at the television: *Or you can clean up your diet, and stop eating garbage!* That doesn't work, but hopefully you will listen and avoid this problem.

Wheat and dairy products are the main causes of arthritis, celiac, lactose intolerance, skin conditions, acid reflux, gas bloating… and the list goes on and on. If you don't believe what I am saying, stay away from all dairy, wheat, and processed food products for two weeks, and I can guarantee you will feel better on all levels.

If you frequently get sick, that's because your autoimmune system is compromised. We are nothing but a huge mass of cells. On a cellular level, we need proper nourishment through vitamins, minerals and proteins. By eating garbage food all the time, you block cell receptors making it impossible for the cells to absorb nutrients and stay healthy. Instead, you are releasing toxic free radicals that actually attack us from a cellular level diminishing our ability to heal and fight off infections. When you eat a proper and balanced nutrition plan full of natural foods, you stay strong and healthy.

Exercise

Exercise also improves libido on several levels. Many men need drugs such as Viagra and Cialis to be able to perform, when this is due to poor blood flow and circulation throughout the entire body.

This can also be caused by eating foods high in omega 6 fatty acids found in most manufactured oils such as canola and corn oil. The acids cause a buildup in the arterial walls restricting blood flow. Exercise and good nutrition will also solve this problem, which is better than taking a pill that causes loss of vision, headaches, and other undesirable side effects. And, when women are self-conscious about their bodies due to weight gain, the last thing that they want is to be intimate. Once again, eating well and exercising will eliminate this feeling by making you look and feel sexier, therefore building your self-esteem.

These are just a few things that good nutrition and exercise can cure. I believe 95 percent of what ails the U.S population is food and lifestyle related, and avoidable. And, much of science is saying it too — that we can control what ails us. They call that "modifiable risk factors." If you want to try a program guaranteed to work and make you feel better, I'm happy to talk to you and work with you.

46

STEP ONE: MOTIVATE!

When asked what I do for a living, the first word that comes to my mind is — *motivate*. I try to show off all the positive aspects of living a healthy lifestyle, while making people more aware of the negative effects of not having one. While many health and fitness experts are extremists and spend lots of time protesting against large companies making junk food, from a personal perspective, I feel my job is to lead by example and educate people so they do not support and eat these products. We are seeing the government step in to begin making changes — food labeling, sugar content modification, GMO management, etc. Companies will be *motivated* to change when we no longer buy their products. By sharing information, scientific data, and giving good examples of healthy living and working with individuals on their personal fitness plans and goals, I hope I am able to motivate anyone who is interested in living a fit, healthy life. As we do our job on a personal change basis, we will impact global change as well.

So — here's where we start!

M — Mind must be in it. This is where it all begins. You have to realize that it is time for a change. Your mind is the will power and your heart is the drive. You need to play the scenario over in your head that you are taking the first step. This step is up to you and is the only way you will improve your situation. Sound mind — to build a sound body.

O — Overcome all fears, excuses and obstacles. You are not the first person to make a change for the better and you won't be the last. Set goals that are attainable then progress from there. When this happens, you are on your way and nothing will stop you.

T — Take the first step. Buy some workout clothes, sneakers, join a gym, hire a trainer, recruit a partner. Whatever it takes to get you started on your path. You will find that this is the toughest step, but once you start feeling the benefits you will realize you did the right thing.

I — Integrate health and fitness into your lifestyle. Now that you started, make it your routine, just like eating and sleeping, make fitness part of your life. I'm not telling you to be obsessive about it, but do make it a high priority. Schedule it as a regular activity. And give it priority on that to-do list.

V — Value your existence. What are you worth healthy versus sick? Realize what you are worth to your family and career. If you say I am too busy with work and family to exercise, ask yourself these questions, "What if I have a heart attack, become diabetic, get sick or become obese? What do I do? What does my family do?" Taking care of yourself is money in the bank, and an investment for your later years. When you take care of you, everyone around you will benefit.

A — Appreciate how simple a healthy life can be. If you are eating whole foods, and exercising on a regular basis, I can guarantee that you are feeling better. If you are exercising properly, I guarantee you are moving better, standing taller, looking better, and performing everything in life at a higher level. Appreciate this — you worked for it.

T — Turn away temptation. It's around every corner. Don't totally deprive yourself of treats and cheating once in a while, but don't make it a habit, make it a rarity. I love sweets, so when I want cake or a cookie, I buy one piece or one cookie and eliminate the temptation of going back for seconds. Do not buy these treats in bulk. Don't keep them in your house.

E — Exist at a different level. People who do not live a health-conscious lifestyle see people who do as an oddity because we use food and exercise as our path to what I consider a functional existence. You will more than likely no longer need to rely on OTC drugs to alleviate joint pain, asthma, or indigestion. Your behavior associated health risks will decrease dramatically, your waistline will get smaller, you will have more energy, and you will definitely elevate your mood. You will exist at a different level. Call me odd if you want — but I'll be at the top of the hill waiting for you.

47

SUCCESS STARTS WITH GETTING ON THE RIGHT PATH

In order to be successful at anything in life, you need to follow the right path that will get you there. Along this path you will make some mistakes, encounter some distractions, and meet obstacles you must overcome. You may come to several forks in this path that require you to make decisions, and you will need to give some thought as to which road to take. The road to health and fitness is no different than the road to financial success or anything else worthwhile. So before you set out on this journey, you must make sure you are carrying some ION'S in your pocket or you will deviate from this path, take the wrong direction, and never reach your destination.

Inspirat-ION: one must be inspired by something or someone to want to seek out this journey. Even when you are doing it for health reasons, someone you care enough about inspires you to stay healthy; or if you have a person you want to emulate, that is an inspiration to get moving. Whatever reason you have to take care of yourself began first with a thought, an idea, and an inspiration. Keep that thought top of mind.

Motivat-ION: the first one gives you the idea, but motivation is needed to carry out the task. This is "the one" that grabs you by the collar, pulls you off the sofa, and pushes you into the gym. "I'm the mud run that's a month away, or the buddy that tells you he can bench more than you; I'm the guy in the movie with the abs who your girl gasps at when his shirt comes off. I'm also the guy hanging around your waist making the scale cry. So basically, I'm responsible for whatever gets in your head and says c'mon man — let's do this."

Determinat-ION: *de·ter·mi·na·tion* — noun —

> 1. firmness of purpose; resoluteness. — "he advanced with an unflinching determination." Synonyms: resolution, resolve, willpower, strength of character, single-mindedness, purposefulness, intentness;

> 2. the process of establishing something exactly, typically by calculation or research." determination of molecular structures"

That about says it all. In order to succeed you must be determined NOT TO FAIL.

Execut-ION: once you are inspired, motivated, and are determined to carry out your goals, the final and deciding round is execution. You can imagine being in shape all day long, be motivated to join the gym, actually have the determination to make time to get there, but all those noble deeds will be undone if you do not execute properly. You only get paid for results, regardless if you are at work or at the gym, the only thing that will propel you forward is results, and the only way to get results is through proper execution.

So let's go over these steps to success one more time. First, we get inspired and that plants the seed. Then we need to find a way or reason to start this task, whether it's a fitness routine or trying to improve your income, something must motivate you. Your follow through will depend on how much determination you have and how much drive and passion you are willing to invest. The end result will be based on your way of executing the situation. Put these IONS in place and you will pave your way to success.

48

Take a Deep Breath.
Start Again

I like to drive fast. I am not reckless, but when I get behind the wheel, I am not going for a Sunday joy ride. I have somewhere to go, and I usually have a short time frame to get there. So as I was driving in the snow this week, I was forced to slow down and in a lot of instances, had to come to a halt. I expected this, and although not happy about all the hold-ups, I stayed calm and shrugged it off. I turned up the music, slumped into my heated seat, and enjoyed the white blanket and the snail's pace that the state was moving in. Why? Because it was all out of my control, and getting aggravated would have been a complete waste of energy. So, I started thinking and putting it all into perspective. I told myself that this was a temporary setback, and when the snow melted, things would be back to normal and I would be able to speed up again. Then I started thinking deeper, and realized that most setbacks we encounter in life are temporary, and with the right mindset, we can overcome them and move on. Here are a few common setbacks we will encounter in our lifetime and how to overcome them.

Stops & New Starts

Falling off your nutrition / clean eating plan can be frustrating, especially if you regain some of the weight you worked hard to get off. These setbacks can be caused by holidays, summer cookouts, vacations, extra overtime at work, school, and numerous other things. It happens to all of us. The problem is that some people let minor or manageable setbacks completely derail their goals. They give up, and everything previously worked for goes away. Instead of stepping back, figuring out a solution, marking a new deadline on a calendar, and creating a plan of execution, some people self-sabotage, or use setbacks as an excuse to quit. This approach will always create more work when you try to get back to where you were. So, next time you fall off the clean eating wagon, tell yourself that the best way to overcome this setback is to assess the situation and figure out a way to get back in your routine. If you are on vacation and there isn't any healthy food you can eat, make the last day of vacation your deadline for bad eating. Hit the ground running as soon as you go home. Unpack and hit the market. Holidays come and go, and so should the eating celebration. Instead of letting your careless eating continue till March, then scramble to get fit for the summer, make changes ASAP. Working too much overtime at work? Can't get out to eat clean? Either bring food with you, or know when this busy season ends, and set a goal to get back to your program. My first year in business took a toll on my training. I was so busy, I didn't get to work out enough, but I always ate clean and found ways to stay active. Now I have a coach and I set appointments, and pay for it. I am not up to full strength, or feeling invincible again, but I am feeling stronger every week. Whatever it takes, just know that this is a temporary setback, and you can fix it if you want to, and try hard enough.

Injury / Sickness

Although there are some injuries and sicknesses that can unexpectedly disable you, there are many instances where people let these occurrences hold them back longer than they should. Many folks milk injuries or bouts of sickness way too long, and the longer you stay away from your fitness lifestyle, the harder it is to get it back. I have examples of two different people who had major injuries, but had different mindsets, and the difference in their recovery time is amazing. A guy I work with suffered a major knee injury. One that could have left him off his feet for eighteen months, but instead he had the mindset that this injury wasn't going to defeat him. Granted this guy is an athlete, and athletes have a more competitive demeanor than most, but he was back in the gym working out in three months. He could have (without judgment) stayed on his back for a year, but instead took the high road, realized this was a temporary setback, and got himself back in working order, quickly! On the other hand, I know someone that had a similar injury, and he allowed it to alter his life. He used pain as an excuse to be miserable, lazy, and get himself addicted to pain killers. He didn't do the proper rehab, and it has taken years for him to recover. Instead of this being a temporary setback, he let it bring him down — for years.

We are all going to encounter temporary setbacks in life. It's a fact, and there is no way to avoid it. The thing that will be different is how each person handles them. You can see it exactly as it presents itself, as temporary. And, you can choose to look at the positive light at the end of the tunnel, or you can decide to live in darkness. We will all get sick, injured, have accidents, so don't adopt the "why me?" attitude and spend your days wallowing in pity and grief; instead figure out a way to get yourself back on track. Get up, brush yourself off, and take back control of your life. It's yours to live — or ruin. You decide.

49

THE RIDE OF YOUR LIFE

Are you willing to accept everything the way it is? Or, do you think you can change things that are undesirable in your life? Sometimes life stops you in your tracks. I was at a funeral last week for a friend who lost her dad unexpectedly, and I listened deeply to the words spoken by the priest. I respect people's faith and beliefs, and feel that everyone has a right to worship or believe in a higher power or spirit. So listening to the words of the priest, and hearing him read certain passages, I started to think deeply and interpret what he was saying. Some words were comforting, but others seemed to be words to get us to accept the tragic loss of a loved one, and this is something I have a hard time doing. His words may be beneficial to help us cope, but I can't accept that the untimely loss of a loved one was "meant to be" or that it is "what this higher power has planned for us."

My friend who just suffered the loss of her father decided to come to the gym more often, joining a fitness challenge promotion I ran that month. I can truly say that my heart was heavy when I watched what she is going through.

We all deal with things differently, some talk it out, some lash out, some bury their pain in alcohol and drugs, and others survive by being tough and resilient. My friend decided to come to the gym more to clear her head, and got support from our Fit Body family. I say to do whatever it takes, without hurting others, to get through a situation you can't control, but never accept things you can alter — like your health.

The words in your head become your reality

Playing messages like this over and over in your head become fatalistic thought. "I don't have time to work out, so I'll never reach my goal." "My parents are overweight." "I have a family history of heart disease and obesity." Or worst of all, "I have bad genetics." These are all terms of accepting who you are even when you are not happy with yourself. But they are just cop-out terms. This is unacceptable to me because I feel that 95 percent of our population has the ability to be fit and healthy if they really want to be. In life we always have choices. We can accept who we are, or we can strive harder and become who we want to be.

Change is a choice you make

When someone who is overweight tells you that they are happy being that way, they are lying to you. I don't believe they are happy — they are accepting the fact that they have zero motivation and drive to be better. When someone gets sick and goes on medication instead of changing their nutrition and lifestyle, they are accepting the fact that they will always be sick, and giving in to the revolving door of medicine. Other people use their kids as a reason for being out of shape and unhealthy. They accept the fact that their life is no longer theirs, but belongs to their kids. My come back is, "I have lots of fit parents in here AND they work and have careers, plus there aren't any kids that want fat and unhealthy parents, nor should you put the burden on them of taking care of you when you get older." After I come back with that, they usually agree with me.

As I said earlier, with most instances in life, we do have choices. We cannot decide how *long* we are going to live, but we can decide *how* we are going to live. So, my question to you is, are you satisfied with yourself? How you look? How you feel? Your livelihood or income level? If you can truly answer yes, then you are living a good life. If you answered "no" or "not really" or "not enough," then you have two choices: get up and make some positive changes, or just sit down and accept things the way they are and live the life that's less than what you wanted. Life is not a dress rehearsal; there is no "take two." Time is our most valued treasure and can't be re-wound or refunded. So, live your life and spend your time wisely, because as another friend of mine says, "you're going to be gone for a very long time — make today the day you start on the ride of your life."

50

TIME FOR INDEPENDENCE!

Today is July 4th — so I feel that it is appropriate to write a column about freedom and independence. Yes, we are considered a free country, and yes, we are an independent nation under no one else's rule. But on a personal level, many of us are not free as we are dependent on others to survive.

I am not talking about the prison population; it's obvious that they aren't free, and I am not talking about children who depend on adults — also obvious. I am talking about the people who are captive and dependent due to their own poor choices, or bad genetics, or who are uneducated due to their socio-economic upbringing or circumstances. I am talking about the people addicted to street drugs, or dependent on pharmaceutical drugs to make it through the day, and I am talking about the obese people and those who struggle with eating disorders, or are captive to food addictions.

Now I am not one to sugarcoat things, and I am a firm believer that if you want something bad enough, you will go out and find a way to get it. I also know that nothing comes easy, and anything worth having requires motivation, discipline, and execution. I have zero sympathy for lazy people who do not try to succeed in life, or people who feel entitled to a good life but who do not want to work for it, or those who blame everyone else for their short comings.

But there are people who are misinformed, and they make bad decisions and poor choices because they were manipulated or given the wrong information. I feel sorry for the people who put trust in their financial advisor and are then taken of their life's savings. I feel badly for the people who read labels on food packages that make health claims, but are being taken-in by false wording, only to make them fatter or sicker. Big food manufacturers lie and spend lots of money marketing their lies. I feel badly for the people who visit a doctor and get put on medication that can cause worse side effects than the original problem, only to find themselves in a vicious cycle of medicine trying to cure aliments caused by the drugs taken for a previous symptom or ailment. I also feel bad for someone who joins a gym to better themselves and gets hurt, or hires a bad trainer and doesn't get any results, but spends a lot of money and wastes a lot of time.

All the reasons mentioned above are a big part of why I opened Providence Fit Body Boot Camp. It was so I can help more people become free from obesity and disease, and help more people become independent from food addictions and the pharmaceutical drugs that control their lives. Nothing makes me happier than someone smiling after they step off the scale and their weight is down, or when someone tells me their doctor cut their meds in half because their blood sugar is under control. Yes, folks, big news flash — proper nutrition and exercise will make you free and independent. But how, you may ask?

So here are a few ways

You join my program that guarantees results. After a few weeks, you get stronger, leaner, and start receiving compliments from friends and co-workers. This frees you from poor self-esteem issues, and you start seeing yourself in a different light. You now like looking at yourself in the mirror again. You start a proper nutrition program, and within weeks your body is no longer inflamed from poor quality foods. Your joints feel better because your arthritis is under control, and you are not dependent on a bottle of anti-inflammatory pills to make it through the day. When I work with older adults, they are ecstatic when they can open a jar on their own due to improved grip strength, and they feel safe and more independent without the help once required to conduct simple tasks in their lives. Or there is the person who is able to return to work sooner after an injury, because they strength trained prior and recovered better, and now has independence from being unemployed. So being able to live alone, feeling better about how you look, boosting self-esteem, having more energy and drive to get tasks done during the day, are all ways that exercise and nutrition can help you gain personal freedom and independence. If this sounds good to you, give me a call and let's get you on a program. In the meantime, just say no to the hot dogs and pasta salad this weekend, and be free from abdominal bloat and feeling tired and lethargic. It's Independence Day — and there's no reason why that can't be about not only our country, but you, too.

51

BE THE CHANGE
YOU WANT TO SEE

S ome people have it, others don't. Some stay motivated all the time. They always arrive to work on time or early. They are always prepared for their day. They never miss a workout, always eat healthy, and never let their health diminish because they stay in shape year-round. Others don't have the interest or motivation, and it takes a wake-up call from the doctor or hitting rock bottom to turn things around and gain the strength they need to make a change.

The good news is that we all have the ability to make changes that will result in self-improvement. Many people just need to change their daily habits, and create a positive mindset. You have two choices: either do something now or wait until you have no choice. And by then it becomes more difficult.

I prefer being pro-active rather than being reactive, but others don't always see it that way. They wait until they get sick, or can't fit into their clothes before changing their lifestyle. I try to encourage people to get and stay healthy BEFORE this happens.

Sometimes it's a matter of *needing* something, rather than *wanting* something. Many folks need pressure in order to correct the problems they have. I always tell people that I can't want it more than you. This means that I can't want you to be fit and healthy more than you want to be, or the program here at Providence Fit Body Boot Camp won't work.

Are "you" worth it?

The people who are most successful are those who wake up and look in the mirror and say to themselves, *"You* are worth it. I am going to take better care of you before it's too late." It works this way with earning money, also. Some won't work hard or change jobs they hate until they are in debt, broke, or so stressed out they require medication. Then they are forced to step up and make some changes. But others make the choice to not let that happen, and they work their butts off to prevent it.

The fact is that you are not alone, and whatever problems you may have, know that others share your pain. Life is difficult for many of us, and we are going to run into roadblocks that could potentially bring us down daily. Don't let this be an excuse to let things get out of hand.

First, you need to realize the things that need fixing, and if you can't do it alone, get help. Focus on your goals and what you can do to make yourself better. Don't compare yourself to others. There will always be someone who has it worse than you. Don't compare yourself to them. Stop telling yourself, "I'm 50 pounds overweight but my friend is 100 pounds overweight, so at least I'm better than that." This will keep you from accomplishing anything.

Look for positive influence

When setting goals, you need to look up to someone who will have a positive influence on you, not someone who makes you feel content. Someone always has it better. Also, don't compare yourself to them, either. Not only is that discouraging, but you don't know everyone's situation; and what appears great on the outside could be fatal on the inside. Someone could look fit, but have family and financial issues. I know a lot of millionaires, and sometimes I let myself feel inferior to them. But when you look deeper, money is all they have, and that's not the most important thing in life.

I am not a financial advisor, nor am I a therapist, but what I specialize in is getting people both physically and mentally healthy. I do it through movement and good nutrition. I know for a fact that when your health and physique improves, it creates a domino effect in your life for the positive. I also know for a fact that everyone is capable of better health and fitness, and the most common thing that stands in the way is the way we think. Or don't think.

So — THINK!

Yes, think — think about where you are now, and think of where you could end up if you continue the lifestyle you are living. Then think of how you can improve it before it's too late. If it's fitness and health you are after, drop me a line. Remember it's better to be pro-active than reactive.

52

CLAIM
YOUR INDEPENDENCE!

I t can hold you back. It can prevent you from going after your dreams. It can blind you from opportunity. It can prevent you from having fun and living a fulfilling life. It can stress you out and cause unhealthy anxiety in your life. This component that causes so much negativity is a thing called *fear*.

Whatever success you want to achieve is just on the other side of fear. It prevents many from achieving their goals and breaks people down to the level of mediocrity. It could decide the outcome of a competition, or change the direction of your life.

If you are afraid, you are unsure, and when you are unsure, you hold back or retreat. When you are in that mode or mindset, it's very tough to advance or succeed. It's the opposite of confidence in many instances, because when you display confidence, you are in the right mindset and most likely on the path to succeed in whatever it is you are doing. Win or lose, you still come out on top, because taking a chance and failing will build more character and true life experience than never trying anything at all.

F-alse E-vidence A-ppearing R-eal

This is a good acronym because it states the truth. Think back to when you were a kid and all the things that scared you. Were they real? In most instances, our fear was for ridiculous reasons. The monster under the bed, the boogeyman, the dark... Yes, these things are all scary to a child, but are the fears real? Absolutely not. The first day of school, moving to a new town, the first time at bat, the neighborhood bully... These are all things that we all blew out of proportion when we were younger, and we let them get the best of us, for no apparent reason. What a waste of negative emotions!

Now, look at what we fear as adults. Opening up a business. Going to a gym. Breakups or divorce. Sending a kid to college. Yes, all scary things, but when you really think about it in depth, what's the worst that can happen? What is scaring us? With business, you could fail. But if you did the research, and it looks like a winner, don't act out of fear — the fear that will hold you back from achieving your dream. Now, don't get me wrong, being fearless and taking high risk chances isn't bravery, but more like stupidity. We still need to apply common sense to our actions. Lack of fear combined with stupidity can be dangerous. If you do research and it points to a bad outcome — and you do it anyway — you are not fearless; you lack common sense. So don't compare being fearless with being careless.

Going to a gym and making a lifestyle change scares people. That's why I have created an atmosphere here at Providence Fit Body Boot Camp that embraces a community environment so you don't feel like you are alone. Heck, what are you afraid of? Losing weight and looking fabulous? How crazy is that? Yes, the big gyms filled with fancy equipment and loud music can be very intimidating to many, but once you develop a routine, and settle in, you will always be OK. When you come to my place, I make you put your fear on a shelf, and guide you to your goal. Eliminate fear, and success will follow!

Going through a divorce or break up is scary, and a lot of people will stay in a bad situation from fear of being alone. This, too, is a fabricated fear we instill in ourselves, because in most instances, leaving a toxic relationship will open new doors and increase the likelihood of finding happiness.

Sending a kid away to college will scare the hell out of most parents. You all think the worst, but again it's a fabricated fear mindset that stresses us out for no reason at all. In most cases, you are doing your child a favor and opening new doors for them, introducing them to the best times of their lives. You end up looking back and realizing how foolish your thoughts were.

Change your mindset

So instead of always thinking the worst, start to change your mindset and think of the good that could come from the things that scare you. Live your life from a place of power. Remind yourself daily, regardless of what you're facing moment to moment, that you are stronger than anything you are going through, facing, or have to handle. Refuse to operate at the level of the problems or challenges that you're facing! Project yourself into the future, and see yourself victorious as a person who has resolved, completed, and achieved your goals.

Keep your head up and your spirit strong, and continue to develop an achievement driven mindset. Tell yourself that you're going to operate at the top of your game and STAND OUT! Apply your best thinking to the issues before you, and bulldoze your way to the top! You have something special. You have GREATNESS within you!

53

First, You've Got to Want It.

A guy came up to me last week after a presentation I was giving and told me I really tell it like it is, no B.S. or sugarcoating the truth. He stood about 6' 3" and weighed over 250 pounds and said that he needed a little reality check to get him off his behind, and start moving again. Then he said, "Thanks, I'll be here tomorrow."

Well, if you know me at all, you know that I tell it like it is. I rarely use a filter, and people have been known to say to me, "I can't believe you just said that to someone." I always respond with "Why? What did I say wrong?" You see, I'm not trying to insult, criticize, judge, or hurt anyone's feelings, so if what I say doesn't sit well with you, it's because I speak the truth, and the truth can hurt. If you are overweight and out of shape, it's because you eat garbage, and don't take care of yourself. Now who would get offended by that statement? And why? If someone told me that I would be more successful if I continued my education, or I would have more clients if I knew how to sell and run a business better, I wouldn't be mad or insulted by them; I would agree with them and do all the necessary things I needed to do to improve, make changes, and move forward. Instead of taking things out of context and whining or complaining about your current situation, take accountability for your actions and make some positive changes that will improve your life. If what someone says about you hurts, or hits home, it's time to do something about it instead of moaning and groaning about what someone said to you.

I am here to help people. That's my mission, passion, and goal, and I will do whatever it takes to get my people to work with me and follow my path to ultimate health and fitness. I'm not trying to sell a workout or a meal plan. I am trying to convince people to make a lifestyle change for the better, and follow my lead on that journey. Three workouts, three weeks, or even three months isn't enough; incorporating changes and new lifestyles into one's daily life is what is needed.

I do give constructive criticism, and I do hold people accountable. I don't hold hands or coddle. If you need that then it's best not to work with me. I also don't give constant praise for "trying," because I'm one of those people who don't go for giving medals for "participating." Trying is a cute word for failing. You're not working hard enough. If you try — hard — to lose weight and get fit — you will be doing it — not trying to.

Why?
It takes hard work and discipline to reach your goal. One of the first questions I ask people that attend my orientations is "Why are you here?" I ask this because you need to have a purpose and goal in mind before you start your journey. Are you here to get fit and healthy? "Yes" is always the answer. Then we peel back another layer, and I ask, "Why did you choose my place instead of the other gyms in the area?" Is it because you dislike crowded gyms full of intimidating equipment and people? That usually brings a "Yes." Then I explain the steps it will take to be successful with my program. Hard work and discipline. That's the only formula to health and fitness. You need to work hard, have discipline, eat properly,

and avoid eating the wrong things. When, and only when, you incorporate these things into your lifestyle will you see the results.

I'm good at what I do, but I can't want it more than you do. And to be successful, you need to be willing and ready to change. Statistically, we are in trouble as a nation. Obesity, heart disease, and diabetes are skyrocketing every year. People are getting bigger and sicker every day. There isn't a nice way to put it. If you continue to eat processed garbage on a daily basis, and don't incorporate some sort of exercise regimen into your life, you are going down the path to self-destruction. You will become a statistic. It's not a matter of if, it's a matter of when.

54

LOSS IS TOUGH.
STAY IN THE GAME.

Loss is tough. I have had times when I was up financially, and times when I have been down. I was never wealthy, but I was on my way to a comfortable lifestyle in the early 2000's. I made some great real estate deals, then in 2006-2007 it all fell apart and I was close to broke. That time in my life put me in a depression, and it was tough to bounce back. Going in reverse, by the time I was turning 40 was not what I had planned. But that's what was happening, and it happened to me — but now I am going in the right direction again.

If my life was always status quo, then I would never have been on top and would have never known how good it felt to be on my way to financial freedom. Taking the hit made me smarter and stronger and hopefully it will never happen again. Nobody is immune from unknown factors that could change our lives or impact us in a negative way. But there are ways you can lower the odds of it happening to you. For instance, I now have business coaches, a financial planner, and I am less frivolous with spending money.

If you don't have your health...

The same goes for your health and wellness. The worst thing in your life to lose is your health. I came down with some sort of chest and sinus flare-up this week that knocked me out for 48 hours and drained all my strength. One day I was on top of my game feeling great, getting great workouts in, and operating at high levels of energy, and the next day a 4-year-old could have beat me. I am not a dramatic person, and I realized it was not a terminal illness and I would be back in action in a few days, but nonetheless, it killed me being off my game and not being able to perform at my peak level.

Many people don't take good enough care of themselves to know or feel what it is like to operate at peak levels, so when they get sick, it's not as dramatic a difference. If you eat processed crap, smoke, and drink regularly, then you have no idea what feeling great is. I do! I eat healthy, exercise regularly, get rest on the weekends, and it has worked. I haven't had as much as a sniffle in two years.

Like financial disaster, I learned that nobody is immune from getting sick, but you can also decrease your odds of it happening too frequently, because nothing is as important as your health and wellness. During those two days, nothing mattered more to me than getting better.

Take care — of you!

I made sure my team had the business tied down and my clients were getting their workouts in, but beyond that, I didn't care if another dime came through the door. I slept till 10 a.m. on Wednesday and it didn't even stress me out that I wasn't at work. I knew I needed to sleep and rest in order to get better. I thought about getting up and working on my laptop but I didn't because my priority was to get back to full strength. I would rather give zero effort than struggle to do something halfway, and pay a bigger price for it later. So I drank tea and slept.

In conclusion, nothing is more important than your health: not money or any other material thing. I tell all my clients at Providence Fit Body Boot Camp that I focus on health before fitness, and when you start doing the right things to become healthy, your fitness will automatically follow. Nothing is worse than losing your health, even for a couple of days. *Did I already say that a few times?* Well, you can tell what a dramatic impact it had on me this week. My life has been going along pretty well, and I'm telling you this not to get sympathy, but to tell you that I consider myself a soldier and will keep fighting back from everyday setbacks until they plant me in the ground. Millions of people lose money and bounce back and millions of people get sick and recover. There is nothing we can do to fully prevent sickness, but we can decrease the odds by taking care of ourselves, eating right, working out regularly, and adopting a solid base of good habits. If we do that, then we give ourselves the ability to limit the damages. When a setback comes your way (and there will be some) just know that there will be better days, but you just have to keep fighting. You have to stay in the game.

And if you prepare for it by taking care of yourself, you will have the strength to do so, and the recovery time will be much quicker. Then it's time to get back to work and dominate your goals!

55

DO NOT
WASTE WISHES ON
WHAT COULD HAVE BEEN!

Wishing for your past to change is a wasted wish, because it will never come true. You should be exerting your mental energy on something more productive like planning your future.

The other day I uncovered my old high school football jersey. I chose #77 because I always loved the Oakland Raiders growing up, and my favorite player, Lyle Alzado, wore that number. He was a menacing force on the football field, and I wanted to be like him. As I held up the jersey and relived a few glorious moments on the gridiron, I thought to myself, "I wish I had been a better player. I wish I had trained harder, practiced harder, paid more attention to the coaches, and didn't party so much in high school."

wishing for your past to change is a wasted wish, because it will never come true. You should be exerting your mental energy on something more productive like planning your future.

The past is gone

The past is gone and the future is formed by the actions you do today. You can't change the past, nor can you predict or guarantee your future, but you can change your thoughts and actions TO-DAY. And that's what I wanted to write this article about... making changes.

We are all doing something wrong in our lives. Not to the point of committing a crime, or hurting someone else, but things we can change to improve our current situation. You don't need me to tell you this, because almost everyone reading this article (unless you live in denial) knows what they are doing wrong. So my question to you is... what are you going to do to fix it? Or are you even going to try?

Sleep with the moon. Rise with the sun.

Every time I have someone sitting across the table from me, whether it be for a sales consult or a nutrition assessment, they admit that they know something they are doing wrong, and it's my job to help them find a solution. When I tell people they need eight hours of sleep, the response is "I know, I just don't do it. I stay up too late either working or watching TV." Then I try to convince them that sleep is one of the most important factors in health and wellbeing, and that late night TV isn't a good sacrifice for their health. It's all about the choices you make and looking beyond immediate gratification and seeing the whole picture. When you get your eight hours, you wake well rested, rejuvenated, and ready to have a more productive day. You help create hormonal balance by sticking to your circadian rhythm: sleep with the moon, and rise with the sun. You feel better, and are in a better mood. Now what's more important? Getting to bed on time, or watching Jimmy Kimmel? And if it's work you need to get done, you are better off going to bed early and setting your alarm clock a few minutes earlier, and accomplishing your tasks first thing in the morning, when you are fresh.

Another thing I call to people's attention is that they don't get enough exercise. "I know, but I haven't had the time"! So my response is, "But we all have the same 24 hours in a day." If we spend eight hours sleeping, and 10 hours working, that leaves us with six more. 50 minutes of muscle building, fat torching workouts is all you need to energize and invigorate you. In addition, it will get you in better physical condition which creates a domino effect by building more self-esteem, self-confidence and also elevating your mood by raising endorphin levels. Now, isn't that something worth etching 30 minutes out of your day to do?

Recognize your problems; map the solutions

We all deserve a better life. We work hard and stress ourselves out daily. I am no exception, but I keep looking for ways to improve so I can coach you to do the same. The first step is self-awareness. You need to recognize that you are doing something wrong. Then you need to write a list of solutions. Then analyze the list and decide which task you can handle yourself, and get help with the rest. Not motivated to work out? That's what guys like me are here for. Call me, walk through my doors, and your problem is solved! Eating too much junk food? Keep a journal, and eliminate the things you know are harming your health and adding unwanted weight.

Realizing what you are doing wrong, and the positive effects of changing those habits, should be incentive enough for you to want to make a change. Do it for yourself. Start by making one simple change at a time, and before you know it, you will be living a healthier and more productive lifestyle. Don't wait until it's too late. Don't wait to sit back and look at your past and "wish" you would've done things differently — because you can right now by making changes. Today! Remember, wishing the past would change, is a wasted wish.

56

25 Tips
to Avoid
the Holiday Bulge

During the holiday season, if you are like most people, you are freaking out a bit. If you're not careful, all that holiday stress will show up around your waist. But don't worry, because the bulge stops here! I put together my TOP tips to keep the "bowl full of jelly" belly at bay.

1. Start your day strong and healthy — not with garbage cereal or a sugar filled coffee drink.

2. Curb your appetite. Drink a glass of water before every meal. It will help you fill up faster and help you eat less.

3. Slow down. Eat slower and taste your food. It takes about 20 minutes for your brain to recognize how much is in your stomach. It is a good idea to take a break after you eat to lessen the temptation to go for another serving!

4. Stay active. Exercise with your family and go for a walk or jog outside! We have normal scheduled classes Saturday so come in and stay on track!

5. Keep a food diary. Tracking everything you put into your body will help to point out your weaknesses. You will then be able to focus on limiting your intake of certain foods and spot when you missed a meal. What you measure you can manage!

6. Choose to eat clean 80 to 90 percent of the time. Eat more protein, vegetables and fruit and healthy fats like nuts and seeds. A handful of almonds or a freshly sliced apple is a great snack to curb your hunger!

7. Don't go anywhere hungry. Try to arrive at holiday parties having already eaten something healthy. That way you won't be too prone to digging into high-calorie party foods. Also, bring a healthy option to a holiday party!

8. Maintain portion control. Pay attention to how much you put on your plate. Use smaller plates. Moderation is one of the most important elements in weight control — especially at holiday parties!

9. Choose water over alcohol. Drinking water in place of alcohol will keep you hydrated and keep your energy level high. Also — it is amazing how quickly calories in alcoholic drinks can add up! Try not to drink your calories for the day!

10. Don't eat things if you don't like them. Sounds simple enough! If you put it on your plate and it doesn't taste as good as you thought, why eat it?

11. Don't give up! Falling out of habits you are trying to accomplish for a few days, DOES NOT mean your effort is hopeless. Simply acknowledge that you "slipped up" or ate poorly and get back on your plan. New day, new start!

12. Exercise on days you eat a holiday meal. Try to get a workout in on the days you know you will have a big holiday dinner. Your metabolism will be running higher and chances are you will choose better foods!

13. Decide how many drinks you are going to have before the party. Choose light and clear alcohol over dark, and alternate between an alcoholic beverage (if you are drinking) and water (same goes for soda). This cuts hundreds of calories!

14. Eat more vegetables. Try to fill half of your plate with vegetables.

15. Wrap up leftovers immediately. If you wrap them up, you are less likely to eat them mindlessly when you are already full.

16. Say "no" to keeping unhealthy leftovers in the refrigerator. These foods will tempt you! It is best to keep your kitchen full of healthy foods so when hunger strikes, you don't have high calorie options to choose between.

17. Use the dirty napkin trick. When you want to stop eating throw a dirty napkin over your food.

18. Throw the snack plate away. When at a party, if the plate is plastic, toss it. If it is a dish put it in the sink. The longer you hold on to your plate, the more you will eat.

19. Have a protein shake or healthy bar snack before you go. If you are heading to a party or other gathering you can have a "clean cheat" with a healthy and awesome smoothie, so you don't pork out at the party.

20. Split dessert with somebody. This way you will only have half the calories!

21. Set goals for yourself over the holidays. Read them first thing in the morning, throughout the day, and before bed. Share these goals with somebody to help you stay accountable!

22. Brush your teeth. Brush your teeth after you eat so that you won't continue eating. Or, keep chewing gum with you and do that instead!

23. Leave the kitchen. Don't hang out by the food table at home or at parties. Too much mindless eating!

24. If eating out, put half the meal in a take home box before you start eating. This will help you with portion control!

25. Make a workout calendar for yourself! Commit to a certain number of days per week for exercise. Cross them off with a marker to show your progress. The more stress you have, the better you will handle it when you work out regularly.

If you have any questions, or I can help you with your fitness and health goals, please be sure to let me know. And — Happy Holidays!

57

CONSISTENCY = SUCCESS

Getting to the gym won't get you in shape. Eating a clean breakfast won't make you healthy. Packing all your meals and scheduling your workouts on your calendar isn't going to help you achieve any of your fitness and fat loss goals. What the hell am I talking about? I tell my clients to do this stuff weekly, so what gives?

True, I do tell people to do this stuff, but none of it will work UNLESS you make it a habit. So, today's topic is *consistency*. All the things I just mentioned are the perfect formula for getting fit and healthy... prepare, eat clean, and exercise. BUT these are things you need to structure into your lifestyle, and do on a daily basis.

You need to create good habits to follow daily. Doing this stuff one or two times a week isn't going to cut it. Exercising and eating clean for a month isn't going to do it either. You need to practice your good habits every day in order to achieve the success you envisioned for yourself.

I see it all the time. People start out gung ho, and then the workouts and results taper off, and in some cases the results achieved diminish due to lack of consistency. And to me it's a shame to let hard work go to waste. I know it's hard to stay motivated year-round. I also dread working out sometimes, but I make it a priority, and have made a commitment to myself not to miss a workout. Since I am the owner of Providence Fit Body Boot Camp, I can get a structured workout anytime I am free during the day. This gives me no excuse, and I am always satisfied that I got it done.

I dread working out sometimes, but I dread being out of shape and in poor health even more. So, decide what would be worse — dragging yourself to the gym, or tacking on a few extra pounds, feeling like crap, and being disgusted with yourself.

Just like your fitness routine. You "gotta" do it and do it daily, or things won't change. As much of a pain as it is to prepare your meals and drag yourself to the gym, it needs to be a part of your life. Design new workouts every day, make them 30 minutes long, and get a nutrition consultation, and supply them with an easy to follow meal plan. Because we know creating to and sticking to good daily habits is tough, we eliminate every excuse not to. That is how my Providence Fit Body Bootcamp operates.

You can't ever stop doing it, and in order to get better and more efficient at things, you need to make them habits and be consistent at following them. I try to make it a habit to read a few pages of something daily. Although a few pages aren't going to make me a genius, it will add up over time, and the knowledge will continue to grow.

Yes, just like exercise. You aren't going to reach your goal in one or two weeks, but if you keep doing something positive and take steps every day, you will reach your destination. So, even if you belong to a gym, and shop at Whole Foods, know that you need to make this part of your daily life. Continuously try to create good habits and follow them. If you keep taking one positive step daily, the tasks you dread will become so habitual, you won't even think about it, you will just "get it done."

Remember, action and consistency = results

58

Everything's Changing How Are You Doing?

This week I had a bittersweet moment. It was my last time training the seniors on my high school football team. Most of them had been with me since I started four years ago, and it was great watching these kids develop into great athletes. This was the toughest group to watch go, because I had trained them the longest, and I really enjoyed working with them. This is a good example of how personal growth can sting sometimes, but at the same time something positive has happened.

This week begins the last month of the year! How exciting! Many of us are busy preparing for the holidays, year-end celebrations and tying up loose ends. Many people also get depressed this time of year, and I think a big part of it is due to one simple thing... CHANGE.

Year-end and the holidays remind us how things have changed and what will continue to change in the new year. But many of us don't like change and have a hard time adjusting. We'd rather keep things as is. But, if things and times don't change, then progress doesn't happen.

Yes, it's hard to know I won't be training these senior football players anymore, but a good number of them will carry on and play college ball. This is an example of a positive change that is happening to many lives. From them, to their parents, to the coaches, and to the teachers who helped mold young impressionable lives — all positive change.

I'm at a point in my life where I embrace change. I tend to jump in with no hesitation believing that failure is never an option. I love learning and growing and challenging myself to accomplish things that are truly out of my comfort zone. I wasn't always like this. I used to like to leave things the way they were; but several years ago, I learned that in order to improve at anything in life, you can't keep doing what you are doing and expect growth.

So, after years of workshops, self-help books and tapes, I learned to make changes. If I can do something better, or if I find a product that's better and more efficient, I'm all over it and willing to sacrifice the comfort of what I know versus the fear of the unknown to make improvements in my life. The world is constantly evolving and changing for the better, and if you aren't willing to make changes, you will miss out and be left behind. One thing that never changes ise the formula for ultimate health and fitness.

And here it is:

Drink clean water: The population has switched to soft drinks loaded with sugar and chemicals that is contributing to the demise of the human population. If you made this switch, hit rewind and go back to drinking water only.

Eat whole unprocessed food: When we made the decision to genetically modify our food, and have a diet of primarily processed manmade garbage, the instances of death and disease began climbing. Before you know it, 75 percent of the population will either have diabetes, cancer, heart disease, or become obese. So, if these items consume your nutrition plan, let's make a change back to eating off the land, and consuming only whole and organic foods.

<u>Sleep eight hours:</u> Most of us live such a high-paced life, we lack sleep. Folks work longer, and watch way too much TV, and miss out on their sleep. There are too many reasons to list here why rest is important, but muscle recovery and a strong immune system are both by-products of solid rest. So, if you aren't getting enough sleep, it's time to make a change in your routine, and get to bed earlier.

<u>Exercise 30 minutes a day</u>: If you aren't doing some kind of movement based exercise daily, it's time to change the routine and get it in. What, no time? Providence Fit Body Boot Camp runs 30-minute sessions guaranteed to get you results. We run 11 to 13 sessions daily, so the excuse about time is irrelevant. You need to move and stay active in order to become fit and healthy, so find the time to get this in.

<u>Change is tough:</u> It's scary and uncomfortable, and can be sad at times, but we all need to do our best to embrace change and move forward. Some changes are forced on us, like the change my team will be making. It's part of the process for people to grow and move on. Your parents have felt it, or will eventually, and that's not a bad thing. Yes, it's sad to say goodbye, but when you look at the road ahead, it's necessary because the future holds promise.

Some changes need to be made voluntarily, like a change in lifestyle if you are sick or out of shape, or change in a career when you plateau and stop growing, or changing a relationship that's toxic. Yes, it's hard but living an average, below average, and unhappy life is a lot worse. "I have never done that before" or "that's not how we usually do things," are two of the most dead-end statements you can make. Those are statements sure to halt all personal growth.

Folks, the world is constantly changing and we all need to embrace change in order to grow.

Find a few things in your life that need to improve in order for you to become happier and more content. Then focus on making small changes daily and creating good habits for yourself. When change occurs that you can't control, find the positives and focus on that, and don't worry about the way things were. Think of how things are going to be.

59

HELLO, WEEKEND...
DON'T BLOW IT NOW

Ahhhh… the weekend is finally here. You get up every morning, some of you regularly exercise (maybe you attend my 5:25 a.m. sessions), then you're off to work with your healthy lunches and snacks planned for the day. You made it through five days of laser sharp focus, planning and execution of daily tasks that include everything from making breakfast to packing your gym bag before bed, so you are ready to go the next day. You worked hard all week and you deserve a pat on the back for taking care of yourself and taking care of business. So now the weekend is here, and I have some advice for you.

DONT BLOW IT NOW!

Don't let the weekend be a reason or excuse to fall off and regress. You worked too hard to let this happen. You bet I look at social media. I see your posts with the doughboys, and steins of beer on your table surrounded by nachos and pizza, and those *ooey-gooey* recipes. And my advice to you is — don't do this to yourself.

I am not saying you need to be perfect. Hell, I look forward to that extra hour of sleep, and the pizza, and the dessert that I allow myself on the weekend. But everything in moderation.

Yes, it's nice to not be on a schedule, and to have some free time to enjoy yourself. But don't let this be an excuse to destroy yourself and diminish all the hard work you put in all week long.

You see, I don't feel like going backwards, and regressions to your goals are "living a little" or "rewarding yourself." I feel that a week of hard work and preparation should end with a few relaxing days to yourself so you can rejuvenate and be refreshed for the next week.

It's a time to do things you like to do, and not worry about time or schedules. It's not a time to do damage to your body and sabotage your will power. Remember, it takes a 3500 calorie deficit over a week's time to lose one pound of fat. So, if you ate healthy all week, and blow it in two days, the scale will not give you favorable results on Monday. Therefore, all your hard work gets minimal results, and to me that's a shame. Yes, every workout is beneficial, and every time you walk into the gym, you will get a little stronger and feel a little better, but as I say over and over again, it's the nutrition component that will decide success or failure when trying to improve your health and aesthetics.

There you have it folks. The decision is yours. You can either stay focused all weekend and have a small cheat here and there and stay in damage control mode, or you can go into it with reckless abandon and suffer the consequences come Monday morning, and all week long.

So, before you go for round two from the bar, or eat that second doughnut, remember all the burpees, pushups and squats you did all week and ask yourself… is it worth it? We got this, folks. We have one life to live, so let's get it right!

60

HOW DO YOU SPELL SUCCESS?

I have received several comments on several social media posts from friends, family, and acquaintances congratulating me on my success. Although I always like getting positive feedback, I feel the word success is a very subjective term. I feel this way because I do not see myself as being fully successful — yet. Though I have a vision of what success should look like.

Yes, I have helped hundreds of people lose thousands of pounds. I get comments from people saying that my staff and Providence Fit Body Boot Camp has changed their lives, the business is growing, and my start-up debt has gone down substantially in the past two years. But I feel like I am a long way from calling myself successful. I still have so much more to learn about business.

I still have a mission to change thousands more lives, and help more people achieve their fitness goals. I feel like I am just starting to climb the ladder of success and it's a long way to the top. I understand that it takes time and a lot of effort to get there, and I have in my head that I will do whatever it takes.

Then I read an email from a guy named Martin Rooney I have been following, and it gave me a new perspective. It went like this:

"Success in life can simply be seen as the amount of your time that you spend doing what you love to do that either makes you happy or have fun! You see, no matter how much money you make or things you have, you are not successful in my book if you are not spending most of your time really happy. I am happy presenting, coaching, writing, training, traveling, and being around my friends and family."

Interestingly, that is what I do with most of my time. Those two statements he made helped me realize that I AM successful to some extent. I love coaching, writing motivational material for my audience, working out, flying to the west coast a few times a year, and spending time with people I enjoy. I am also making a good living doing what I love to do; therefore, I feel somewhat successful.

But it's a big ladder, and I still need to keep climbing. I came up with my own acronym and I want to give you my definition and the steps I feel you need to take before you can truly call yourself successful. Here it is:

S-sacrifice. You won't get there until you make the sacrifices needed. You can't stay up late watching TV and taking the next day off. You have to sacrifice some things you like to do for the things you need to do. If you want success in fitness, you say no to cookies, cake and alcohol. If you want success in business, you sacrifice a day in the park for a day in the office.

U-understanding. It won't be easy. Even if you love what you do, it takes hard work and discipline to achieve true success. Remember what Steve Jobs said, "If you look closely at most overnight success stories, they actually took a long time!"

C-creating a plan. You won't get there by guessing and it won't happen by accident. You need to map out a clear plan to follow, and have an idea of how you will accomplish your mission.

C-courage. You will need to take chances and step out of your comfort zone, and that gets scary at times. Fear will hold you back from achieving your dreams, so you need to develop courage and fight fear.

E-execution. Ideas and thoughts are useless unless you act on them. You will only achieve results from taking action, and taking massive action. Remember, a plan is just words or ideas until you execute.

S-systematic. You need to perform many of the same tasks day in and day out to achieve results. These need to be productive tasks, and need to be improved upon daily in order to create a successful system. Once this happens, things will flow much more smoothly.

S-satisfaction. This is the epic term. This is why I don't feel fully successful. I am not satisfied yet. I have so much more to do, and so many more obstacles to get over. I am close, but not satisfied that I have done everything I am potentially capable of doing. I am happy at the progress I am making, but satisfaction is still a few steps away. It's like someone wanting to lose 20 pounds. Yes, they will be happy losing 10, and people will call them successful when they lose 15. But you won't get full satisfaction until the goal of 20 is reached. I feel like this is a good thing, because in most cases when you are satisfied, you get complacent and progress usually stops. So being a little unsatisfied will keep you actively trying to improve the things needed to achieve your goal.

Success is a subjective term. We all have different interpretations of what it should be because we all have a unique set of goals and visions we want to accomplish, therefore no one person can put a label or give an exact definition of what it is. It is an individual ac-complishment. I feel that all human beings are capable of creating success for themselves whether it be raising a family, losing weight or making lots of money.

We all have it in us to become what we want to be, it just takes focus, discipline, and massive action. You need to set your goals, devise a plan and go after them. The big bonus with becoming successful is that you find happiness and live your passion along the way. When you are happy doing what you do, you've achieved a big element of success!

61

YES, YOU CAN!

s an adult, two words should never leave your mouth again — and those two words are "I can't." When you are a child, those words are acceptable because you are limited to what you can and can't do. *Want to go to a movie? I can't; I'm being grounded. Come over to my house for a play date? I can't, my parents are busy, and I don't have a ride. Have a piece of cake? I can't, my parents are responsible, and they don't let me eat sugar. Let's talk on the phone tonight. I can't, I need to do my homework.*

As a child, we had limitations placed on us by our parents and adults who supervised us, but as an adult, the only limitations we have are the ones we fabricate in our heads and place on ourselves. In most cases, we can do whatever we want, but we don't due to self-limiting beliefs we carry around inside us. So, the words "I can't" should not be part of an adult's vocabulary.

<u>Let me give you some examples</u>

Want to go to a movie tonight? Now, everyone has the ability to achieve this task, so instead of saying — *I can't* — some other options may be phrases like *I already made other plans*, or *I'm tired and need to get to bed*, or *no, I have something better to do*, or *I don't want to go*. These are more truthful answers to this particular question.

We have a meeting tonight at six, are you still going? If this was planned and you say *I can't* you need to immediately change your tune and say, *I was going to, but something more important came up, and I am doing that instead*. Because as adults, we all have the power to dictate how we spend our time.

I can't be a millionaire can be translated by saying, *I am not willing to work the long hours, take chances, or step out of my comfort zone in order to do so*. We all have the ability to achieve success and financial stability, but many of us are going about it the wrong way. When you see someone who's super successful and you tell them *I wish I was like you* — you need to step back and think about what you are wishing for. Success comes with a price, and not everyone is willing to pay that price.

Now let's move on to the fitness spectrum

I can't seem to lose weight. Now here's where I tend to lose my cool. When someone says this to me, I instantly want to say, *yes you can, but you need to stop eating garbage food, and devote yourself to a regular fitness and training program*. You see, the first thing I tell any client that walks through my door is you need to adopt a positive mindset and that all the training and nutrition will not work until you do so. As a matter of fact, I do not allow the words *I can't* to be spoken in my facility because we all have the ability to live a fit and healthy lifestyle, but we have to adopt a few good habits first. It's actually pretty easy.

There are four components to healthy living

1. Eat real food. Stay away from processed man-made garbage, and eat what mother nature intended us to eat.

2. Hydrate with clean water. Every cell in our bodies requires water to thrive, so drink half of your bodyweight in ounces of water daily, and you are good.

3. Sleep. You need rest to regenerate and repair muscle tissue, so get to bed on time and get your eight hours nightly.

4. Move. At Providence Fit Body Boot Camp, we run 30-minute sessions all day long, so you have plenty of opportunity to squeeze a workout into your busy day.

YES, YOU CAN

Folks, as adult humans, there isn't anything we can't do. It takes a bit of programming, and a lot of positive mindset that can take time, but by implementing small positive daily habits, you will take more and more steps towards the big goal. Start today and incorporate the habit of NOT saying *I can't* during your daily routine. This is your first step to success in any arena. Once you lose the self-doubt and cop-out statements, you will put yourself on that path to positivity.

SECTION TWO

BODY
& FITNESS

1

How to K.I.S.S.
Your Way
To Fitness

KISS stands for "Keep It Simple, and Safe" — and it is a phrase that typifies my approach. Many people today who are trying to be fit think they have to do ridiculous things to get results. And, if truth be told, there are many fitness instructors who will play right into that concept. I'm here to tell you that you don't need to be complex with crazy amounts of equipment and complicated techniques.

There is so much confusion in the fitness industry, and so much good (and bad) advice and so many theories. With proper training technique and guidance, based on research and education and a whole lot of common sense, you can have a workout program that is holistic for your body, healthy for you, and will accomplish your long-term goals. It will become a way of life, not a dreaded "have to" that you begin finding ways to avoid, and not a compulsion that you "must do" and overdo. Here are some quotes I hear from people on a regular basis, and my responses to them.

I do hundreds of crunches every day

Rarely do I, or have clients, do crunches because when you flex and bend something repeatedly on the same plane, it will get weaker and eventually break. This is not good for the spine or the posterior spinal stabilizers. It also creates an imbalance by making the rectus abdominal stronger than the spinal stabilizers. And thinking "simply" again, how functional is it to move repeatedly within such a short range of motion?

I'm going on a no carb diet

I don't subscribe to this method for weight loss or general health. Based on research that your brain and muscles function on glycogen, I feel that eliminating all carbohydrates puts you at a disadvantage for endurance and muscle recovery. This is especially true after a workout and when your glucose levels are low. I do believe in limiting your carbs to quality sources, such as quinoa, sweet potatoes, brown rice, and legumes. These carbs are fibrous carbs, and are much lower on the glycemic index than processed grains.

I need to lose weight before I start lifting

Doing that would actually slow down the process of weight loss. Here's why: strength training speeds your metabolism. While lifting weights, you are burning calories by contracting your muscles. Lean muscle tissue burns more calories at rest. Thus, by lifting weights, you are burning calories while performing the activity which leads to muscle mass which leads to a faster metabolism.

I had an egg white omelet

But you threw away the part of the egg with the most nutrients! An organic, free-range egg is loaded with beneficial fats and proteins and other healthy compounds such as vitamin D and numerous amino acids. The whole egg is also considered an anti-inflammation food. The white by itself contains about three grams of protein and the yolk has four grams of protein. So you are throwing away more than half the nutritional value for the money you spend on good quality eggs. Eat the yolks — you won't get fat — and they taste great.

I had a great workout — got sick — and can't walk today

This is not an indication of a great workout. Going to the gym, running, cycling or whatever activities you do, you are doing to promote health and fitness. Throwing up after a workout doesn't seem healthy to me. Tearing your body down to the point where you can't walk the next day or are in severe pain isn't the right approach, either. I train myself and my clients hard but not to the point of being incapacitated for two days or vomiting. I want you to feel mobile and invigorated after a workout. You will sweat, shake, and be out of breath, but never sick or in debilitating pain.

I work out and I do cardio every day

To all you work out folks who are having trouble attaining your goals, just step back and reassess your situation. It doesn't have to be difficult. You don't *need* to work out and do cardio *every* day. You don't even *need* to join a gym. And let's talk about rest — real rest — rest that rejuvenates the body, rest your body cannot do its best work without. Stay tuned for a future column on rest.

In the meantime, remember — Just KISS!

2

"FULL EFFORT IS FULL VICTORY" — GANDHI

I t was Monday afternoon, and the high school football team I work with was 3-0. As I approached them at practice, I could see that they were expecting a celebratory talk from me, but that's the last thing I was thinking about. I went over to the group and started clapping. I clapped and said, "here's to a win, fellas" but after about 10 seconds I yelled out "that's enough!" I told them that being 3-0 was no reason to celebrate, due to the mediocre play they were exhibiting. Out of those three wins, only one was hard fought against a tough division team. The other two wins were over smaller, lower division teams that we took lightly, and just squeezed by. We were SUPPOSED to win those games, and we didn't play to our fullest potential. That's where my frustration sets in. We are a great team, with lots of talent, but we are disorganized, and lack drive, discipline, and focus, and that could cost us this season if we don't change our attitude.

Good enough isn't any good at all

Whether it be sports, business, fitness, or just everyday life, I feel that doing "just enough" to scrape by is unacceptable. If you invest time, money, blood, sweat and tears into something, it's worth putting in 100 percent — your all-out effort. When you do this, I think you will

ALWAYS get a better return on your investment. I told this to my team, that it all starts right here on the field. If we don't go out and play to our fullest potential on every play, down, and in every game, someone will come along and blow us off the field. I tell them that if this "just get by" attitude continues when they get older, that they will always be struggling to get by with everything they do. I said that they will live paycheck to paycheck and never accumulate wealth, or create a surplus of money, because "just enough" won't allow it. I feel this way with my clients also. When you join my gym, Providence Fit Body Boot Camp, you are not paying for workouts, you are paying for results. You are paying for leadership and coaching to get you to your goals. You are paying for someone to hold you accountable. You are paying to belong to a community of like-minded individuals all striving for the same thing ... outcome! And when people make a monetary investment in me, I encourage them to give 100 percent. Just showing up isn't enough, and the most important work is done outside the gym. After you invest your sweat and hard work exercising your body, you need to exercise discipline, and eat the right foods, and make sure you are getting enough sleep to recover. I encourage my clients that doing the bare minimum won't cut it, and you have to put in the time to prepare, and execute, to get favorable results. It's harder and requires more work, but the end result is worth it.

It's 100 percent or bust

I not only preach this philosophy to my team and clients, I try to live it myself. I have been running my new business for exactly one year now, and to many it seems I am successful. But not to me. I feel that I am operating well beneath my potential, and that bothers me. It's not due to lack of hard work, it's due to inexperience. I am striving to get better every day. Instead of resting with the things I am doing right, I am obsessed with correcting the things I am doing wrong. I know that when I accomplish this, the return on my investment will be much greater, and I will become much more successful. So, whether it's sports, fitness, or business you are investing in, my advice is to go all out, and give 100 percent of yourself to accomplish your goals. If you do this, you will become unstoppable, you will succeed every time, and the return on your investment will be far greater than if you do something half way.

If it's worth doing, you will find a way. If it's not that important, you will find an excuse! Hard work and discipline are the main ingredients to achievement, and we will only get paid when the work is completed!

3

1-2-3: REST!

All this talk about doing, and now I want to stress the importance of UN-doing. While I believe that every time you work out you need to bring it on hard and train like a warrior preparing to fight gladiators, on the flip side, your body must be able to withstand the punishment, and only two things insure that: rest and nutrition (hydration falls in the category of nutrition).

It is impossible to train with 100 percent intensity if you are injured, sore, unmotivated, or fatigued. Over training elevates cortisol, your sympathetic fight or flight hormone, and elevated cortisol over long periods of time causes your body to enter defense mode, making it tougher to burn fat. It also slows down healing, impairs digestion, metabolism and mental function. So, if you work yourself hard, without attention to rest and recovery, you can end up with a negative result — not a good result — for all your blood, sweat, and tears.

Other problems associated with over training include recurrent injuries like tendinitis, stress fractures, adrenal fatigue, chronic fatigue, amenorrhea (the absence of menstrual periods in women), constant muscle soreness, joint soreness, regression (not making any gains in the gym or on the field), exhaustion, illness caused by a weakened immune system, and irritability.

Take a day off from strenuous physical activity every three workouts, or as necessary. I know there are lots of workout fanatics out there who will say you don't have to do this, that only working out constantly will get results, but we also need to exercise some common sense and pay attention to our bodies. Just like when you feel hunger pangs, you eat, so when you feel overly exhausted and sore, rest.

This is perhaps what makes me different from an average personal trainer, because it's where my holistic training comes into play. My advice is train hard and rest easy. As with many things in life, it's all about balance.

You want to do something that makes you feel good, and relax. If you say intense exercise relaxes you, you are not doing it right. No, doing yoga correctly isn't a "break." Some yoga classes are as tough as any other workout.

So, as I've given advice on exercise, here are my suggestions on rest and rejuvenation:

Take a meditative walk — leave your phone and music behind

Get in touch with yourself and nature, by paying attention to your posture, foot strike, breathing fresh air, and core stability.

Massage

Massage increases circulation which speeds muscle repair and re-generation, increases disease fighting white blood cells, decreases cortisol, and heals the body. And it feels great.

Sleep eight hours

This is tough for some, but you have to make the effort. The benefits of sleep are enormous, including mood elevation and mental alertness. Many of our bodies' major restorative functions like muscle growth, tissue repair, protein synthesis, and growth hormone release occur mostly during sleep. Sleep also lowers adenosine levels in your system. Adenosine levels are thought to lead our perception of being tired. Sleep improves memory, is said to help us live longer, curbs inflammation, spurs creativity, improves performance, sharpens attention, lowers stress, and sleep regulations aids in managing depression.

Spa day

Whatever you can afford to do… do it!

Lay in the grass/hammock and take a nap

Sit around the house

Veg out

Watch a movie or TV — it's OK.

R-elax
E-njoy yourself
S-leep
T-rain harder

4

BACK TO BASICS —
CORE STRENGTH

I heard one of my mentors offer this great analogy: if you lift weights or strength train with a weak core, it's like firing a cannon from a canoe. Think about it! Or I say, it's like building a fortress on sandbags.

I see it daily. People in the gym killing themselves for an hour, then get on some "ab" machine or do a few minutes of crunches, and then go home. Sure, they might look great from a distance, but when you look closer you notice the forward head tilt, the weight belts, the rounded shoulders, etc. These people are guaranteed to acquire back pain due to the lack of core strength and stability.

If you are a golfer or waiter with lower back pain, it's usually due to instability of the core. Having a strong core requires two things: proper nutrition and proper training technique. When your midsection is properly conditioned, you not only look better, you stand taller, lift heavier weights (if that is part of your goal), and perform your daily activities better and with less injury. All core routines should consist of abdominal and lower back training using movements in a multi-plainer range of motion.

When you're out shopping this holiday season, take note of how many companies have their workers wear belts to protect their backs — from the UPS driver to the warehouse people at Home Depot. Wouldn't it be better if they had a proven employee fitness program in place? If we lived as they do in Eastern cultures, there would be many companies starting their day with stretches and exercise to strengthen the core — and improve productivity and health — not to mention attitude and demeanor, all at the same time.

Again, set your goals, and regardless of what they are — bulking up, having less injuries and strain, looking great, or being in your best condition — remember, it's all about THE CORE regardless of what else you do.

5

BACK TO SCHOOL

Throughout my career, I've trained all kinds of people — men, women, young people and older people, from ages 14 to 90. Something I've done for a few years now which is particularly satisfying is to work with a high school football team as their strength and conditioning coach. It really doesn't matter if they are football players, because my training advice would be the same, pretty much, for all age groups. With kids going back to school, being fit and healthy means they'll be better at reducing injuries, be more focused, and have more discipline — all things they'll need to be better students.

Athlete or not, it all starts with basics

Strengthen the core. Condition the body. Eat a healthy diet. Get enough sleep. Watch unhealthy habits. This advice is good for all types of young people — the athletic, the sedentary, the in-between, the boys, and the girls. My observation is that teens in general are awkward. They have weak cores, poor balance and stability, and lack coordination. This goes for athletes with the exception of those who are gymnasts. Part of this is due to poor programming and improper training. I find that they go to YouTube or muscle magazines for their workout direction where there is a generalized lack of attention to core and proper movement patterns. Even on an athletic level, most coaches at the high school level know the game and strategy of the game, but lack resources and time to provide proper strength and conditioning training. The same goes for gym programs — it's often playing a low intensity game that everyone can do, rather than learning about strength and conditioning.

Injury prone without properly conditioning

Teens playing contact sports without the proper conditioning are at higher risk of injury. It's like your spine in an accident without a seatbelt. Another reason for their awkwardness is that they are not fully developed at this age. They are still growing and sometimes not uniformly. Their bones grow faster than their muscles in some cases, causing long lanky limbs with loose, unstable joints. Doing the proper types of exercise is extremely important at this age because their bodies are still developing, and high-risk exercises that load the spine should be avoided until an individual is strong and stable enough to support such activities. Attention must be paid to movements and addressed accordingly. When trained and fed properly, this age group responds quickly to exercise and conditioning. Whether your child is an athlete or not, it is a good idea to give them incentive to, and educate them about exercise. It will pay off in the long run. Girls need to be handled carefully when it comes to eating. I helped a friend's teenage daughter lose 65 pounds by educating her on food quality, then she took over and did it on her own in a healthy way.

The football team didn't win the title last year, but we exceeded the coaches' expectations, and injuries were lower than usual with the team maintaining high levels of energy — and there's always this year. We've already started working out at Providence Fit Body Boot Camp.

I always start by developing a mutual respect between us, and explain what and why we are doing something. Exercise is important at any age, but safe exercise is essential at this age. So, along with shopping for new clothes and supplies, let's get our kids off to a healthy start — it's a holistic approach that makes for smarter kids, healthier kids, and happier families, too.

6

EXERCISE — DISGUISED

I do not have any children of my own, but I do have a nephew that I am fortunate to get to spend a lot of time with. Whether he's my own or not, every male has aspirations to see other males in the family excel at playing sports or performing other physical activities. My nephew doesn't care nor does he have the drive to play any sport. His interests are geared more towards action figures which used to be frustrating to me not because I wanted him to be competitive, but because of health concerns — such as his motor and strength development. But last weekend we went on a rock climb / hike, and I realized that with what we were doing, in addition to his time in the playground, that this kid is getting just as much physical benefit as he would in a baseball or soccer game on a team playing intermittent turns with other players. He climbs, we run. And in the playground, he develops strength on the bars, and works his core on the swing. Perfect primal training. So I came to the conclusion that instead of asking someone to exercise with you, (buzz kill to most), ask them to do a fun activity that will be a disguise for exercise. Here are a few.

Swimming

Plan a leisurely day at the beach, then create challenges in the water. "Hey, you think you can swim the length of the beach?" Or race to the ropes and back. Swimming is such a great full body workout, that you do not need to do much to really feel tired. Another fun water activity at the beach is body surfing. Walking or running back in against the current will wear out even the most conditioned person in a short amount of time. So, get off the blanket and into the water for some exercise — oops — I mean fun.

Biking and kayaking

These are both fun activities that will torch some body fat in the process. The only drawback is that they require equipment, but today you can rent, so you don't need to buy. And, you can do either alone or with people. Both ways are fun so it's a win / win for you.

Hiking

Back to the topic of hiking. This requires some decent shoes, bug spray (please use organic), snacks and water. There are lots of places here in New England that offer some challenging trails and nice places to hike. Lincoln Woods State Park, in Lincoln, Rhode Island is close to me, so I enjoy the convenience of their great trails, but when time isn't a factor, the options are endless. There are many resources online where you can find good hiking trails, and even mountain biking trails.

For children

It's as simple as going to your local playground, or taking a soccer ball and finding a patch of grass. Whatever you decide to do, make sure your activities this time of year are outside to not only breathe fresh air, but to absorb all the vital vitamin D we have been missing due to lack of sunlight. Enjoy the outdoors, and keeping it simple and staying active while having fun will promote better health.

7

DO YOU HAVE
GOOD S. E. X.?

What's the best and fastest way to achieve your fitness goals? Add SEX to your routine. SEX stands for **S-trength, E-ndurance training,** and **e-Xcellent eating habits**. These strategies will allow you to reach your fitness and fat loss goals faster and more efficiently than any other gimmick or quick fix on the market today. You must incorporate these three elements into your routine in order to have long term health, fitness, and vitality. This is not a quick fix, but by adding SEX into your lifestyle, you will create ever-lasting results. That's why the components of my programs at Providence Fit Body Boot Camp incorporate all three. You see, the key to fitness and health is to lose body fat and build muscle. It's a simple formula, but not easy to achieve. It requires a lot of hard work and consistency to be successful, and it won't happen overnight. Let me break it down for you in a little more detail.

S-trength training

The only way to build strength is to do resistance training. You need to overload the body by creating more resistance than when it's in its natural state. This could be from lifting weights, using resistance bands, or creating it with your own body such as doing pushups or body weight squats. This method stimulates new muscle growth, therefore making you stronger. It also speeds up your metabolism. More muscle equals faster metabolism, allowing your body to torch fat and calories faster and more efficiently, even at rest!

E-ndurance training

The best way to build endurance is by performing high intensity interval training, or HIIT training. This is also the most effective way to burn the most calories in the shortest amount of time. You accomplish HIIT training by doing short intense bursts of exercise, followed by brief periods of rest or active recovery movements. The reason this is so effective it that it ramps up your heart rate, and lowers it periodically, thus causing your heart and lungs to expand and contract more rapidly helping them to get stronger and able to handle a higher uptake of oxygen causing you to build endurance. Steady state cardio like walking or jogging where your heart stays in the "target" zone actually makes your heart and lungs work at a lesser capacity, rather than making them stronger. Therefore, if you want to build stamina and endurance, you need to train accordingly; and if you want fat loss, pick up the intensity.

X-cellent eating habits

You have heard it all before… you can't out exercise a bad diet… abs were made in the kitchen… BUT IT'S ALL TRUE!!

In order to achieve true health and fitness, your eating habits need to be excellent. This means that you need to eliminate all the processed garbage and manmade foods from your diet. These types of foods will not only add pounds to your waistline, but this type of food will make you sick. Anything in a package that was manufactured by people in lab coats and safety glasses is not fit for human consumption. Factory farmed meats and processed foods assembled using GMO ingredients will cause all kinds of bloating, inflammation, and digestive disruption. This causes a domino effect, because when the digestive tract is inflamed, it causes hormonal imbalances which makes it impossible for our bodies to utilize nutrients and function properly. When you stick to an organic diet and eat quality foods harvested in a sustainable manner, it allows your body to function better, and in turn, you'll feel better. When you feel better, you will have more energy which will allow you to train harder, and the end result will be you looking better. Other important benefits are that your skin will look better, your joints won't ache, and your digestive tract will eliminate waste and toxins making for a stronger immune system. Remember you are what you eat, and you are what the animal you are eating ate, so stay away from processed dead food, and eat things that are alive and healthy.

Remember, if you want the best results and you want them quickly **S-trength, E-ndurance training,** and **e-Xcellent eating habits**. It requires a lot of hard work and consistency to be successful, and it won't happen overnight, but anything worth working towards isn't usually easy. So, there's your homework — get to it!

8

ETIQUETTE IN THE GYM?

Yes, gym etiquette is a real concern — and it's lacking in most gyms. I know you go to the gym to sweat and get down and dirty, but there are a few things we can do to make it a nicer, and safer, experience for all. I'm not saying you need to wear white gloves and a bow tie to work out, but some simple courtesy goes a long way, especially during peak hours, when things get crowded.

Unplug

One of my biggest issues in the gym is the cell phone. I understand that phones do many things, but when you are at the gym they should play music only. Really folks, let's disconnect for an hour and focus on the task at hand... exercise and intensity. If you are that important that you can't turn off your phone or email for one hour, maybe you should reschedule your workout times to a time when you can turn off, because answering the phone zaps intensity, and without intensity, your results will be non-existent. It's also bothersome waiting to use an area or a machine when the person is sitting around texting and holding up progress, and it is most annoying trying to focus when someone ten feet away is arguing on the phone. Remember that there is equipment and moving parts, and a gym can be dangerous, so let's be considerate of others and for safety reasons, leave your phone in the locker.

Get to class on time

When I'm doing group instruction, I must explain the importance of punctuality, especially in cycle class or a class that requires equipment and weights. First, you compromise on your warm-up and this is an important part of the workout. Besides that, it is dangerous to start adjusting your bike or set up your area, when others have started moving. Finally, you have the distraction factor. It isn't the end of the world to me if you are late, but what of the others who made the effort and arrived on time? It can be annoying and distracting.

Hygiene

Now let's talk a little about hygiene. Being the cold and flu season, this area should not be overlooked. I have seen many guys leaving the men's room without washing their hands. Seriously? I encourage my clients to wash their hands after every workout. Wiping down the equipment is always a welcome courtesy. Trust me, nobody wants to jump on a bench with a puddle of sweat, or a wet circle from one's head dripping off of it. Take 30 seconds and give it a quick spray, the next person will greatly appreciate it. And while many employees at the gym are mothers, they're not yours, and even if they were, they'd tell you — let's pick up our toys when we are finished. A lot of people feel that paying for a membership entitles them to a personal butler. If you use a piece of equipment, it is easier for the next person to find when it gets put away or re-racked to its rightful place, so please put your stuff away. Finally, if you are sick… stay away! You might think you are being rough, tough and cool working out sick, but you are not only taxing your immune system even further, making recovery time longer, but you are spreading germs to everyone in the building. When it's cold outside, and you have a heated room full of sweaty people, you get an incubator for germs, so please think of your fellow gym goers and keep your germs to yourself. Walk outside if you absolutely need to work out. Germs won't spread as quickly in the cold, and YOU will feel better. Or just rest and recover.

We go to the gym to improve our bodies and de-stress from the days' events. We are not looking for more stress or to get sick. Going to the gym should be a pleasurable experience for all, so if everyone does their part and follows a few rules of etiquette, we can all have an enjoyable workout, stay safe, and stay healthy.

9

EXERCISE HAPPENS FOR A REASON

I started working out to get bigger and look better. When I started in the fitness business 20 years ago, I remember when people would work out to drop a few pounds or get ready for beach season. Fast forward to today and it seems as though more people start exercising due to high blood pressure, diabetes, heart disease, and obesity. Sometimes it's a life or death situation to lose weight and become more fit. Whatever your reason to start or continue to exercise, here are a few more reasons many people don't know about — but might just inspire you to get started...

Exercise increases your sex drive

First, exercise not only makes you feel more desirable, it stimulates blood flow, which releases endorphins that release testosterone and other hormones. Second, you will have a better self-image and that enhancement leads to a greater sex drive. A big part of better sex is feeling sexy. Research shows that people who exercise have an improved body image over people who do not exercise. Being more comfortable with your body leads to better and more relaxed sex.

Exercise makes you smarter

Studies have shown that exercise releases brain chemicals that help with the retention process of new information. The reason is when you exercise, your blood pressure and blood flow increase, which in turn shuttles more oxygen through the entire body — brain included. It raises your focus for up to two to three hours afterward, so it is advisable to work out just before a test or presentation so you will peak when you perform. On a more scientific level, it makes the hippocampus super active, and when you rev up these neurons, cognitive function improves. This pattern works better with regular exercise, because the benefits can quickly recede. So be regular with your exercise patterns, not hit or miss.

Exercise aids digestion

If the food we eat isn't digested properly, a whole lot of problems can arise in the body such as gastrointestinal issues, acidity, acid reflux, heartburn, constipation, bloating, and even bad breath. This is why healthy digestion is probably the most important element to your health. If you can't utilize good nutrients, and eliminate bad bacteria, you end up sick, diseased, and overweight. During exercise, your heart rate and breathing increase, thus stimulating muscles that support the digestive tract, which in turn makes it more active and efficient.

So what will be your reason? Find the motivation that works best for you. If you don't have the motivation and drive to start it yourself, come to Providence Fit Body Boot Camp and I will get you going. Working with a coach will get you there more effectively and efficiently. If one of these inspires you to get started, then go with it. But remember, ultimately it is your health that is at stake, and that impacts all the people around you — your spouse or partner, your children, and your family. And it impacts your ability to earn a living. Being healthy helps you have a positive outlook in life; you're more likely to be happy, in general.

We all need to keep moving — the rewards just keep adding up — so, start now and let me know what motivates you! Leave me a message on Facebook or Twitter… and I'll share your motivation with others. We're all in this life together — let's make it a healthy one!

10

FIT AT ANY AGE

Throughout my 30s, all I heard from my non-fitness friends was, "wait until you turn 40! It's all downhill from there." But I had friends in their 40s who were running marathons, competing in body building competitions, and challenging me at mountain biking. Well, here I am now — at the age of 44. I'm fitter, faster, more mobile, and the healthiest I've ever been. Maybe I'm not as strong as I was, but I am a lot lighter. Why is this? For one, I have another 10 years of knowledge, experience and muscle maturity. I also have developed better eating habits.

The 20s

Let's look at someone in their 20s — that usually youth-driven, full-of-adrenaline person. If they are training, more often than not it's for reasons other than being healthy and fit. I was a bouncer in a nightclub, so I wanted to look big and intimidating. I packed in pasta and pancakes and trained with reckless abandon, including lifting heavy weights.

The 30s

Those in their 30s are outwardly focused—concerned with family and career, often working ridiculous hours, eating lots of less than optimal food including fast food, getting minimal rest, and chasing the American Dream. It can be a time when you are putting your own health low on the priority scale, missing workouts more than making them, even if you are working out at all.

The 40s, 50s, and beyond!

So, then you hit your 40s. You probably are looking at 10 years or more of your kids' leftovers—the mac & cheese, those chicken fingers… you're looking at them right around your mid-section. Add to that a couple of drinks a day hitting your liver, experiencing lower libido, and have adrenal fatigue in your blood. Your kids are in school, and are becoming more self-sufficient. So, you look at your life and make the decision to get your fit life back—now—or to start for the very first time. I promise it's not too late to be 40, fit, and in fantastic shape.

Start with these tips:

Eat better. Avoid man-made processed foods. Make the effort to prepare your meals for the day. Eat a healthy breakfast, lunch and snacks to ensure your metabolism keeps burning all day.

Move more. Anything helps—stretching, walking… Strength training with proper technique builds muscle and helps fight flab.

Relax more. Your body REQUIRES it for repair and rejuvenation. Get massages, eight hours of sleep, etc.

Although not necessary, it might help to have a trainer in some capacity who can keep you on target and moving forward.

It's your time—now! You'll reap the rewards long into the years ahead, reducing disease risk, preventing injuries, and looking great, too. Approach the years ahead in your best shape ever.

11

"MOVING IT..." INDOORS

So you don't like big gyms, can't afford small private training studios, and it's getting too cold to do your thing outside? I guess this means it's time to take the winter off from exercise, right? You can gain ten pounds, lose some muscle mass, and get depressed and de-conditioned, so you have to resort to frantic, unhealthy ways to get it back in the spring. Or, you can spend and purchase a few items that will give you a great workout at home, regardless of your fitness level.

My motto is and has always been, "no excuses." You can achieve your goals regardless of your situation. Time, weather, space or finances are no longer acceptable reasons to neglect yourself or your fitness after reading the following advice.

First, we need a spot to perform your fitness routine, one that you can leave set up, ideally. Basements and garages are ideal spots to create a place to work out. I like these choices because the floors are concrete and you can move around without disturbing others and do various exercises without shaking the house. If you do not have the option of either of these, a spare bedroom or even your living room will work.

Next, you'll need to buy a few things — tools to make your routine fun and challenging. I can get and give a great workout by just using and performing body weight exercises such as squats, lunges, push-ups, planks, and various plyometrics, and add progressions to all, but it is nice to have a few pieces of equipment, too. So here's my list of suggested items to purchase, and a few additional suggestions.

1. *Swiss balls or stability balls.* A great way to add balance to your routine. You do not need a lot of space to perform exercises on these. Some great moves are the supine ball roll, supine bridges, elevated feet planks with knee tucks, wall squats, and supine hamstring rolls. You can purchase a top-quality ball for about $60.

2. *Med balls and slam balls.* You've seen them in old school boxing gyms. They come in different weight increments, and can be used in moves such as abdominal twists, sit-ups, and any range of motion exercises such as squats and lunges, to add weight and movement to any exercise. Jam balls do not bounce when slammed on the floor or against a wall, so standing, kneeling, and half kneeling chop / slams are a great way to work the core and stabilize the spine. Prices range from $15 to $35.

3. *Rubber bands* are a great addition to any exercise routine. Made popular in physical therapy programs, these can take the place of expensive cable machines. They come in different resistances so they can create a challenge to all. Exercise such as rows, chest flys / presses, shoulder presses, raises, rotator exercises, and resisted rotations can be done on different planes with different resistance just by shortening and lengthening the band. You can anchor to a pole or door or piece of heavy furniture and add even more variations. A great versatile "must have" for about $15 to $30 each.

4. *Jump rope* (you'll need ceiling height and a solid floor, of course). This is a great way to get a little cardiovascular conditioning while working on your coordination and footwork. Jumping rope also stimulates your calves and shoulders, and forces you to have rhythm. While jumping, maintain good posture, keep your abdominals tight, and vary your footwork by jumping on both feet, one leg, alternate legs, and increase speed. All this for $12 to $20.

5. *Bosu Balance Trainer*. Popular right now. This looks like a Swiss ball cut in half, with a platform on the bottom. Very versatile tool for conditioning the entire body. You can use it for single leg training techniques, squats, lateral movement, and is durable enough for jumping jacks to reduce impact. Flip it over dome side down for pushup and plank variations. These go for around $50 to $65.

If you want help locating equipment, you can go to my website at www.fitnessprofiles.net. Click on the "Perform Better" banner, and you'll see everything you need to know about the equipment mentioned here. A heavy bag is a great inexpensive tool to train and relieve stress, but you need a sturdy place to anchor it. Cable machines are adjustable so you can train every body part, but they are also expensive and cumbersome. Start with what you can and make progressions along the way.

So... just because the weather is getting chilly, and you need to start moving indoors, don't give up your fitness routines. Remember — we're in this to be fit for life — not for just half the year. If you can join a gym, great, and even if you can't, put together a little home fitness area. Before you know it, all the members of your family will be asking you what to do with this piece of equipment, or that. And that is the goal — to pass on a fitness regime that everyone can be part of. It doesn't have to cost a lot.

There's no excuse for a sedentary lifestyle. So, look around your home and set up your own area that will serve you well, and come Spring, you will not have to start all over again; you'll be good to go back outdoors.

12

PUMP YOU UP!

After writing over 20 of my first blog posts, I found myself on a Thursday night with a Friday deadline looming before me, wound up from teaching my spin class, and wondering why this week's focus wasn't coming to me. I was looking for a fresh idea, an inspiration to write, so I thought about a few encounters I'd had this week. The first was a friend who talked about how good it feels when you get in more than three workouts in a week's time. Then, there was my colleague at the gym — the "beast" we call him — who told me that he was bummed out that work was busy and he had missed the gym all last week. I reassured him that you couldn't tell he missed a beat, and he replied, "but I notice — and I feel it." I knew just what he was talking about. Finally, there was my client who I hadn't seen since Thanksgiving, and hearing her tell me how she felt so much better after our session today. Then, this week's topic hit me.

I found the number one most important reason to exercise...

Not for health, not for aesthetics, not for performance, and not for longevity — but because it makes you *feel good*. Both physically and mentally you just feel good after properly performed exercise. Physically it gets your blood pumping, lubricates your joints, and stimulates endorphins.

Endorphins ("endogenous morphine") are endogenous opioid peptides that function as neurotransmitters. [1] They are produced by the pituitary gland and the hypothalamus in vertebrates during exercise, [2] excitement, pain, spicy food consumption, love, and sexual activity, [3][4] and they resemble the opiates in their abilities to produce analgesia and a feeling of well-being.

In other words, they elevate your mood and give you more energy.

And let's not forget the "pump" you get after a bout with the weights, or the clean feeling of fresh air in your lungs after an outside workout. And the best physical benefit is that your posture improves as your core gets stronger, which makes you stand taller, alleviating many aches and pains.

Mentally it takes away the stresses of the day

If you have been sitting in one place all day, your mind needs to unwind, and working out can put you in another place. When you are working out your main focus is on breathing and lifting with proper form and not the laptop you left in the car. It also builds your self-esteem. Thinking that you are looking better makes you feel sexier and helps build confidence. If you are doing cardio, you can let your imagination run wild. Put on some great tunes, and be a beast! Or, just meditate and go for a walk.

Whatever your choice, just do something that gets you up and moving, gets your blood pumping, and puts your mind at ease. You will feel better. If you don't believe me, ask someone else who exercises, they will give you that confirmation.

13

FIT FOR LIFE... IS AGELESS

I have been asked numerous times by different people, about what I specialize in, and I tell them that I don't have a specialty. I like to make everyone better. I have an age range of clients from 14 to 87 and I enjoy training all of them for different reasons.

Youth groups are challenging

Kids have vastly different abilities. Some are natural athletes, some are built like stick figures, and some have weight issues at an early age. This is an extremely important time in the developmental process, both physically and mentally, so it needs to be approached with caution. On a physical level, bones and joints are still growing, so caution needs to be taken that they don't do permanent damage when exercising. Loading their bodies with weight needs to be progressive and incremental. I would never load a bar on a teen's back and have them squat, for instance. You should wait until the growth process is over to avoid any spinal compression issues. Form is also crucial and needs to be perfect, otherwise you are drawing a roadmap for dysfunction and injury. I have seen fathers in the gym pushing their kids to lift heavier than they should, or performing high-risk maneuvers, and it makes me cringe. Their intentions are great, but their knowledge of body mechanics and movement patterns isn't, so hire a pro to help your teen. It will benefit them for a lifetime.

On an emotional level, it is tough to deal with fragile emotions and body image issues because you don't want teens taking things to extremes such as overtraining or over dieting which can lead to eating disorders. Therefore, I think it is best to educate kids about nutrition based on health and performance goals more so than aesthetic goals. That way they can focus on getting stronger faster while the looking good part just happens, and they are not stressing or taking drastic measures for the wrong reasons.

Middle aged is a transitional time

Those in the 40 to 65 group are in an interesting time in their lives — whether they have kids going to college, a divorce, career changes, or discovering a medical problem. I notice a lot of people wanting to make changes to get their life and body back. Due to maturity and common sense, this crowd usually understands what they need to do, but bad habits and lifestyle are so addictive that starting a new routine can be difficult. Once we get on track nutritionally, I find it only takes a few weeks to get someone in this age group moving properly, showing strength gains, and feeling better.

It is extra rewarding at this age because they feel and move like they did in their 20's. Just by doing body weight exercises, and a few simple core-strengthening moves, their posture improves and this can alleviate lower back and knee problems. Then we start incorporating some strength training, people are amazed at what they can do, especially people who were once athletes. Because with proper cues and techniques, their muscle memory lets them bounce right back into fit form.

I also stress that this group eliminate any kind of pounding on the body, such as running, jumping, etc. unless they are training for a specific event. People actually love the fact that I can get them fit and healthy without long treacherous bouts of cardio exercise. At this age, any bouts of continuous movement at the same pace — moving in the same plane — will cause overuse injuries, or at best, waste time and get nowhere. I see it all the time, people doing the same routine year after year, and suffering from pain and plateaus. This is why it is important to vary the routines and train the whole body as a system, so when we enter the next stage in our lives, we can feel and be ready to leave the masses behind and be vital and healthy.

Seniors

My 86-year-old client is always saying, "If I knew I was going to live this long, I would have taken better care of myself." And I tell her that it's never too late to show improvement as I persuade her to do her dead lifts and squats. Yes, that's right, squats and dead lifts for an 86-year-old woman. Chair aerobics and one-pound weights will not help improve balance, strength, and stability for this population. Let's not forget that senior bodies need to move, push, pull, and lift, just like the rest of us, only slower and with some modifications. This is why all the same rules apply, just with a more conservative approach. Most of the workout should focus on balance and movement by simulating everyday moves — getting in and out of the car, putting stuff in overhead cabinets, using the facilities, getting out of bed, etc. — all the while creating a little resistance, and mildly taking the client out of their comfort zone. We then focus a portion of the workout on strength and resistance.

You need to pay extra attention to this population to not overdo it. Watch their facial expressions, listen to their breathing, and if they ask for a rest, let them have it — immediately. Remember that everything they do is something more than what is done at home. Always follow the first rule as a trainer to "do no harm" especially with this population. When they can bend and touch the floor, lift something overhead, perform tasks that make them feel independent, they feel great, and we feel great knowing how much we improved someone's life.

Fitness IS ageless. It's a constant cycle of assessment, proper technique, and adaptation. Remember what my 86-year-old client said, and look at the long life ahead of you — you're getting fit to live long, and live that long life as healthy and without injury or disease as you can. You'll thank yourself for it in your senior years, and at every stage throughout your life.

14

FITNESS
AND NUTRITION —
SIMPLIFIED

At my gym, we do one thing, and we do it better than anyone else. That one thing is to get you results. There is one question you need to ask yourself when you sign on to any fitness program, and the question is,… Will this place help me achieve my goals and get me results? Not, "How nice are the locker rooms?" not "how many TVs are there?" not "How much fancy equipment is packed into the place?" not "How nice is the décor?" not "Will they give you a wedge of lemon in my water?" and not "Do they sell fancy stuff in their pro shop?" None of that matters if the place doesn't have proof that the program works, or isn't willing to guarantee you results. WE DO!

We don't do it with fancy, trendy equipment. We don't do it inside fancy mahogany walls. We do it by incorporating basic, non-electronic, hand-held equipment like battling ropes, med balls, dumbbells, suspension trainers, and bodyweight movements. We provide coached, 30-minute sessions of high intensity interval training or (HIIT) workouts, and recommend you attend 3 to 5 times a week. But that's just half of the equation.

Nutrition

The other half is something you need to do once you leave the gym, usually the hardest part. And that's your nutrition program. It's not a diet, but a lifestyle you need to incorporate to be successful with ANY exercise program. We provide every member with a blueprint of how you should be eating on a day-to-day basis, and the folks who follow it are guaranteed results. It's simple, but not easy. We make nutrition easy to understand, but you need to supply the discipline and will power to succeed. You eat clean, healthy food that tastes good, and you eat frequently throughout the day. I don't ask you to worry about all the scientific philosophy that goes into nutrition, so you won't be confused. I provide you with simple tips so you will succeed.

Here are my top three tips:

1. *Eat quality food.* The quality of your food is just as important as the amount of food you eat. Good food raised on sustainable farms, without pesticides and antibiotics, is essential to good health and vitality. Your body will absorb the nutrients more efficiently, you will avoid any kind of digestive inflammation, and you are helping out the environment and avoiding cruelty to animals. If you are NOT paying attention to these issues, you are supporting farms that treat their animals unethically and are polluting our soils with harmful chemicals, as well as wiping out necessary insects and organisms that contribute to our closed organic cycle.

2. *Being prepared is essential to your success.* If you fail to prepare, prepare to fail. You can't just wing it on every day basis and expect to eat healthy. When you pull up to a drive thru, chances of getting a quality meal are slim. If you need to go into a convenience store for lunch or breakfast, you will be eating some form of processed garbage that will either hold back your results or put them in reverse. Take the time to prepare your food for the day. *You* are worth the time, and your results will show.

215

3. *Stay hydrated*. Your muscles require water to thrive, and your body needs muscle to get lean. A general rule is to drink half of your bodyweight in ounces of water every day. A good way to make sure you get enough is to buy a case and keep bottles in reach everywhere you go. Keep it in the car (weather permitting) keep it in your office, bring it to the gym, and drink some before every meal. If you are concerned about frequent trips to the lavatory, don't be; that's a sign that things are working properly and your body is eliminating toxins.

So there it is. At my gym, we provide you with this simplified approach to starting out on your health and fitness journey. So, start by finding a fitness program that will guarantee you results, and then incorporate a nutrition plan that is simple and healthy. With a combination like that, you are guaranteed to succeed.

15

FITNESS OR FOOLISHNESS: ARE YOU WASTING YOUR TIME?

* Do you log hours and hours of cardio per week?

* Are you eating nonfat processed foods?

* Are you sore for days after exercising?

* Do you train to total exhaustion?

* Are you starving yourself?

* Do you waste money on gimmicks?

This is most people's interpretation of fitness. If you are doing these things and not making any gains or feeling worse, sore, or relying on painkillers and anti-inflammatories to make it through the day, it's time to change.

The answer is as simple as eating quality whole foods and doing the proper amount of exercise. *Fact:* You cannot out exercise a bad diet. Eating processed foods whether they are low-fat or not will actually make you fatter because most of these foods are higher on the glycemic index causing a rapid fluctuation in blood sugar, thus making your body store fat rather than burn fat.

Strength training is the key to any fitness regime. When you build muscle you burn more calories — period.

Decide on your goals: lose weight, improve golf, play with your children or grandchildren, look better at the beach. Then give yourself enough time to achieve these goals and seek advice from a qualified professional.

Fitness: It's a noun! The condition of being physically fit and healthy. The quality of being suitable to fulfill a particular task or role.

GET FIT FOR FUN

Now that it's nice out, you're thinking to yourself, "I don't need the gym, I'll walk outside. I can ride my bike outdoors. I'll lose weight that way. When summer comes, I'll paddleboard — and swim — instead of going to the gym." I hear this every year about this time, and if you are someone that says or thinks like this, you are making a big mistake.

Exercising outdoors isn't enough. Running, cycling, gardening, and paddle boarding are leisurely fun activities. They are not a substitution for a full body workout. You hear it all the time, heck you may even have said it yourself, the nice weather is here so I will start walking after dinner every night or do some outdoor activities that are going to get me in great shape. Well, you have it backwards! Outdoor activities do not get you in great shape — they *require* you to be in good shape to perform properly and to avoid injury. While walking will burn some calories, it doesn't build muscle. Actually, while everyone is encouraging walking, and yes, it's a good thing to add to your fitness mix, walking is just a little more strenuous than sitting on the sofa. You will lose some weight because you are creating a small calorie deficit, but will gain it all back next winter if that's what your fitness program looks like.

Look at all the seasonal warriors out there who yoyo from winter to summer. Now look at those who work out year-round and you will not notice a drastic change in weight gain from season to season. Why is this? Because when you stay active consistently, you build and maintain muscle mass which raises your metabolic rate giving your body the ability to burn more calories all the time, even at rest. Now don't take this the wrong way, I am a huge advocate of the great outdoors and think you should spend as much time out there as possible. Just don't use it as a substitution for a complete body workout and fitness program. For instance…

Biking: I am a big mountain biker. To me it is one of the toughest activities I do. And there are some intense road cyclists out there who log huge mileage. Both activities burn tremendous numbers of calories and train your heart, lungs, and legs like nothing else, but that's it. What about the upper body, and lower back, and core muscles? See where I am going with this? When you are hunched over for extended amounts of time, your hip flexors shorten, and your lower back muscles get overworked and over stretched. Both are recipes for low back pain. You also do minimum hamstring work while working the quadriceps extra hard, creating imbalances throughout the body. Even though you do not develop strength in the upper body, you require strength there to allow you to ride more efficiently. The only way to achieve this is through resistance and mobility training, and neither can be done sitting on a bicycle.

Running: People who love to run hate talking to me on this subject because I do not advocate distance running, only sprinting. Here's why. Some of the pros of running are that it clears your head, relieves stress, and burns more calories than walking. And some of the cons are that it causes ankle, knee, hip, and lower back injuries due to overuse or doing a constant motion in the same plane in a repetitive manner for an extended amount of time. Running causes unnecessary pounding and lots of impact to the body, and unlike sprinting, it makes your body adapt and become more efficient, rather than challenging your heart, lungs, and respiratory system like sprinting does by elevating your heart rate on an interval basis. Many of you get off the sofa in the spring, lace up the sneakers, and start your running program. To do this without abdominal / lower back and knee and hip stabilization work first this might earn you a trip to the orthopedic specialist.

Kayaking: This activity will challenge the arms, back, and shoulders on a conditioned athlete, so if you are not conditioned, this activity will seem like torture. I never train people in a seated position due to the fact that not many activities require an exertion of power while seated, but this is an exception. In order to do this, and feel OK after, you must maintain proper posture and have decent shoulder and thoracic spine mobility. If you don't, you will find yourself slouching while you paddle, thus causing poor power output, as well as compensation in other areas of your body such as the neck, cervical vertebrae, and scapula. This sport should not be done for extended periods of time without a strong core, and good shoulder stability / mobility otherwise you will be sore for days afterwards.

In conclusion, I do not recommend these activities being used as a way to condition or get yourself in shape, but as a way to actively enjoy the great outdoors. And I certainly don't recommend doing these if you aren't in shape. There is only one formula for getting fit, and that is strength training, cardiovascular conditioning, and proper nutrition. You need to build muscle and burn body fat, and the only way to do that is to use the formula described above. I know that when the weather is nice, being indoors to workout is not that desirable, but here at Providence Fit Body Boot Camp, you get an intense full body workout in just 30 minutes and we guarantee results. In my opinion, that's the perfect solution — get a great workout and not waste any valuable outdoor time, and be in condition to excel at fun activities.

I signed a new client who confessed she had been an avid runner for years but it broke her body down, and after just three weeks of boot camp, she feels tighter, toner, stronger, more mobile, and more injury-free than ever before. But don't just take my word for it, stop in and see for yourself how a great training and nutrition program can change your life. Have fun outdoors, but don't do it to get in shape. Stay in the gym year-round, and you will feel the benefits.

16

FIVE THINGS TO ASK YOUR PERSONAL TRAINER

1. **<u>What kind of training do you have? Are you certified?</u>**

A good trainer should continually seek training and be networking with others in his or her field. You want to ask what that training is — what type of certifications does the trainer have? You might even ask when the last new class was that they attended. And, does the trainer have a trainer, too? Many of the best trainers work with others in the field that we can learn from and will push us to our next levels.

Ask them what kinds of clients they have. I work with teenagers with weight and body image issues, athletes trying to improve their sport, the average healthy person, those with injuries to work around, and even the elderly who want to avoid falls and keep their independence. Do you see yourself in the mix of clients your trainer works with? And lastly, ask about nutrition and if they work with clients on food intake and planning.

2. <u>Do I have to join a gym?</u>

Exercise & equipment changes over time, but basics are still what works the best. There's no magic bullet to get fit, no new piece of fancy or funky equipment. I find that simplicity works best, and sure, while it's great to have high tech equipment to help with some of the move patterns, it doesn't have to be complicated. I work with primal move patterns. So, if you can afford a full gym membership, great, but it's not necessary — and it's not an excuse. Trainers should be able to work around this. Many of us rent space in smaller studios and gyms. We can do a workout outdoors, in your basement or garage, in a large room, and at a company site with small groups. Equipment is also something you want to ask about. Does your trainer have exercise balls, resistance bands, that sort of thing to help you get started if you aren't joining a gym?

3. <u>How important is it to have a one on one experience with a personal trainer? Can't I just go to a group class?</u>

I teach group classes, such as spinning, but before you get started on an aggressive plan to be fit, you need that one on one time with someone trained, and someone who is focusing just on you and your uniqueness. Again, the quality of the trainer is important. Some trainers do high-risk moves, but I don't believe in doing those. You shouldn't start lifting weight with a weak core. That's like firing a cannon in a canoe. Once you find someone trained who knows the mechanics of the body, and understands good technique, and good form, I recommend a conservative approach. First, do no harm, is my motto. The importance of the one on one training is that you will not get a standardized program — do three of these and four of those — and a sheet to mark it off as you go around the gym, but you will get an individual plan formulated after a personal assessment, taking into consideration any unique issues such as mobility difficulties, injuries, or age, as well as your personal goals.

4. <u>Is my trainer asking me about what I eat?</u>

The first thing I recommend is to clean up your diet. I always say, "you can't out exercise a bad diet." So, to do that, you need to know what you are eating. Keeping a four-day log of your food can really be eye opening. Trainers should be talking to you about what you are eating, your alcohol intake, and your water intake. What types of food are you eating? Is it a fast food rich diet? Are you eating a lot of preservatives and foods that are not natural? Again, the best nutrition plan is a simple one. Without looking at this, you don't know what fuel you are putting in your body — is it empty calories? Non-nutritional calories? Does your trainer know about nutrition and incorporate that into your sessions? Will your trainer help you by going to the supermarket with you — helping even to clear out your kitchen cabinets? Fitness doesn't begin and end in the gym. If you have better nutrition, you will feel better, and be better motivated for exercise, too.

5. <u>Is this going to take forever?</u>

No, it shouldn't take forever. But lifelong fitness is a way of life. For goals such as weight loss, for instance, I always say that it will take you just 24 hours. 24 hours? Yes, but that is two hours a week for 12 weeks and I'll have you losing two to three pounds a week, safely. And if you need to lose more, we'll just continue until you come to your best weight. The same goes for strength training or increasing flexibility. In 12 weeks, I'll have you moving better, with improved posture, and you'll build and improve muscle mass. So, no, your goal shouldn't take forever — but lifelong fitness is a forever thing that after a while becomes just a regular part of your day. I also talk about my "three-hour goal" program. Every three hours, throughout your day, do something healthy for yourself — have a glass of water, take a short walk, look up a healthy recipe for dinner, check out a gym membership, have a healthy snack, or park your car the furthest from your appointment and walk. These are little things you can do throughout the day. And don't forget to step away from the things that stress you in life and — very important — get some rest.

A last word. Discipline

That's what all good trainers want in their clients. We want you to be successful. After all, your success is ours, too. We can give you the roadmap, but we can only do so much. We ask you to bring the discipline. With that, your goals are attainable and the partnership between you and your personal trainer will be a win-win relationship.

17

HAPPY SPRING — PANIC TIME!

I t's here! It's that time of year. The birds are out early chirping, the sun is up, and it's lighter earlier. The smell of spring in the air, and it is the time we wear less clothing and show more of our bodies when we leave the house. That's all well and good, and we should all be excited about it unless you are not in the condition you wanted to be in this time of year. Now, panic sets in.

The weather is hitting the 70s, and your waistline is still hanging below your belt. The sun is up earlier, and your butt is sagging lower, and when you wave goodbye to someone, your arm is still jiggling after they have driven away. What should I do, you may ask? Is it too late?

Ideally, I do not like to prescribe quick fixes. I believe health and fitness should be part of your everyday lifestyle, and we should be preparing for this season all year long, not just a couple months or weeks before it arrives. But I have a few things you can do to make things happen a little faster, but you need to do these things without interruption, without missing days, and without cheating at all.

It sounds tough, and it is, but you put yourself in this position. So don't get mad at me for telling you everything you need to do to get out of it. No ifs, ands, or buts — you need to do it this way or it won't work, and your mindset needs to be all-in 100 percent. So here goes.

HIIT or High Intensity Interval Training

You will not get the results you are looking for in a short amount of time if you just jog, walk, or stroll around on your bicycle on the bike path. You need to crank up your heart rate for brief periods of time — rest, repeat, and do this for bouts of 30 minutes at a time. You need to do this frequently, four to five times per week. Frequency and consistency will get you much faster results than working out for one-hour periods of time once or twice a week.

By doing this you are elevating your metabolic rate and burning body fat much faster than conventional long bouts of cardiovascular exercise. You are also preserving muscle mass, unlike longer duration / less intense exercise, which will eventually cause a catabolic or muscle wasting effect due to the long periods of movement without replenishing glycogen stores in your muscles. The key to getting fit is to build muscle and burn body fat. When you exercise too long, the opposite happens. Just look at long distance runners compared to short distance sprinters. Sprinters are muscular and aesthetically pleasing to look at, while long distance runners have some muscle in their legs, but lack muscle elsewhere. They actually look like they are starving, thin, and frail.

Resistance training

It is a must for building muscle. HIIT will burn fat and preserve muscle, but it takes weight to build muscle. You do not need to lift weights so heavy that you throw your back out or turn blue in the face, but you need resistance that challenges you in order to build muscle. No, ladies, you won't get big lifting weights, just lean, mean, and toned. There is a very small population of women who do have the capacity to develop big muscles, but a majority of women carry too much estrogen, a prominent hormone in women, as opposed to testosterone, the dominant hormone found in males. It's all about body mass index.

You want to increase the percentage of your body that's made up of muscle, and decrease the amount of fat you are storing.

Lifting weights will enable you to build lean tissue which in turn raises your metabolism and helps you burn fat along the way. Muscle is a more active tissue which will burn more calories at rest than fat tissue will, so resistance training will build muscle that burns calories faster, and your HIIT training will get your heart rate up so you torch more calories per minute. That's a double attack on body fat, and a proven way to build muscle.

I run a program at Providence Fit Body Boot Camp that does all of the above in 30 minutes. We combine strength training with high intensity metabolic conditioning for the fastest possible way to achieve your fat-loss and fitness goals, in just four to five thirty-minute sessions per week. And you're guaranteed to see results.

Nutrition

The last and most important component to reaching your summer-time goal is in your nutrition plan. At this point, with such a short timeframe to accomplish your goal, this part needs to be flawless, and you can't deviate from it — at all! This means no alcohol, bread, processed junk food, or dairy, and a very limited amount of fruit until you reach your goal.

If you do not do all of what I am telling you, you will NOT accomplish your goal. It has to be all or nothing. No moderation, no cheat meals, no "just a bite" of anything that's not on your nutrition plan. If you do, it will bring progress to a halt, even push you back further, and your summer physique will not appear.

To get lean and tight, you need to consume something nutritious every three hours. These small meals need to consist of a perfect balance of protein, fat, vegetables, and minimum amounts of fibrous / low glycemic carbohydrates, such as beans and sweet potatoes. Some examples are two eggs, kale, olive oil, and half a sweet potato, or grilled chicken breast with a half cup of rice, and a salad or steamed veggies. Your meals do not have to be bland and taste-less, just extra clean and full of nutrition.

It might be vanity for the summer that will motivate you — or your career might be at stake if you are a model or in the fashion indus-try. Sorry to be the bearer of bad news, but if you want abs, or to show some arm definition in that sleeveless dress, this is what it's going to take. If you need help and accountability, you can call me and I will keep you focused and give you direction and all the tools you need to accomplish your goals. Keep that image of what you are working towards in your mind, and keep moving toward it — pretty soon it won't be just an image — it will be YOU.

18

PERSONAL TRAINERS AND FITNESS PROFESSIONALS: COLLEAGUES, *NOT* COMPETITORS

There are many people you can go to for personal fitness training. Some also do nutrition. Some don't. Today, I want to address those of us who are in the personal training field. It's a message everyone can listen to, because if you are looking to work with a personal trainer, I suggest you find someone open to learning different things; someone who is actively seeking out additional training and education whose personality will make your training more enriched and professional.

On Facebook, a trainer who I never met, thanked me for NOT unfriending her for posting feedback on my posts. She told me that other trainers had done this when she commented on their posts. Was this straight competition? Or did the trainer take comments as an insult to the trainer's expertise in the field? Are you kidding me?

If personal trainers and fitness professionals feel threatened or are insecure about other professionals' feedback, discussion, comment, or advice, then I think they are missing the big picture in this profession. Granted, some feedback requires dialogue, and even debate, so let's talk about it! We've seen science change just when we think we know something to be true, and I see us all in a fluid learning environment — particularly we can learn from each other. I welcome comments on my social platforms, or by email or conversation. Just back your input with evidence and what you've learned from experience, be open to other opinions whether you agree or not, and use it to your advantage by learning from it. WE ARE THE FRONT LINE, the messengers — the soldiers. We are in the trenches grinding it out to help people live a healthy lifestyle. It is OUR mission to promote health and wellness to people that turn to us for various reasons.

Our battle is not with each other

Our battle is against disease, obesity, injury, garbage food, poor posture, the perceived need for prescription and over the counter medications, etc., etc. We should be uniting in this fight because we are facing a huge enemy, with lots of resources; more resources than we will ever have. Let's face it: none of us invented movement patterns / exercises / or nutrients — our mission is to try to deliver the best approach for the people we train. I am a 20-year veteran in this industry and I still turn to others for ideas and advice. I seek out continuing education in this field all the time, and I find it invaluable because I learn from guest speakers and networking with other trainers; people I think are experts in the field. So let's leave the know-it-all ego at the door (because none of us knows it all), and join together in this fight on behalf of the clients we serve.

Medical professionals, hospitals and rehabilitation centers primarily treat disease and injury

Let's face it, people look to us and listen to what we say and advise, even more so than they do with their medical professionals in a lot of ways. While the medical field is skilled in treating disease, it has been a relatively short time that they have been talking about prevention and lifestyle change. Medical schools don't incorporate a lot of this information — proper fitness and nutrition criteria — into their curriculum. And, of course, a prevention focus is rarely reimbursable by health insurance (though this could be changing). When we work with our clients on a personal basis two to three hours a week, we are given a great deal of confidence in our abilities. So, never stop learning, listen to each other, and critique each other responsibly and respectfully. Always try to learn more and better yourself in this profession. If you take this approach, I believe that both you — and your clients — will benefit!

Growing our profession

I have even helped other trainers who are my direct competitors. Why? Because if a trainer hurts someone, it's bad for the profession as a whole. We enjoy fairly lax regulations and guidelines, and most certifications are easier to obtain than they should be. But, if someone gets hurt, we all suffer the consequences. We need to bond together as professionals to boost this industry to the level where we can bill insurance companies as preventative medicine, instead of waiting for people to be sick or injured and in need of treatment. This will help people who are paying out of pocket, now, for our services. This time is coming — it is the next step in a holistic wellness approach. We can point to acupuncture and chiropractic care that is now reimbursable and held accountable. Why? Because the profession worked together as a cohesive group. Now is the time to network and join forces to get our message heard, not compete over clients. If you are good at what you do, clients will come, and they will stay!

19

IS MORE EXERCISE
REALLY BETTER?

My teen clients are notorious for asking, "What else can I do on my own?" and "How many more days should I be lifting weights?" And they are surprised and mostly disgruntled when I advise them not to do more. My newer clients always ask how many more times a week do they need to train with me to get results, and they too are surprised when I tell them none. You see, if you follow my system you will get results, and my system does not include over doing it so I do not promote extra exercise until you make the proper progressions and you prime your body to handle the load. Not until then do I encourage extra workloads. I request that my clients and football players give 100 percent effort through the workout and it is impossible to do so if you are sore, tired, and broken down. I told an athlete that I would rather be slightly under trained than over trained and I compared it to a steak on the grill, if you remove it too early, you're safe, and can put it back on; but if you burn it, it's worthless.

Recovery is key

The same goes for your body. When you work out too much, several things happen. Your chance for injury increases due to weakened and fatigued stabilizers and muscles. You compromise your immune system. You elevate cortisol levels, causing hormonal disruption and risking muscle depletion. What doesn't happen is results. Recovery is the key to making gains. You will never reach your goal unless it is becoming "skinny fat," or staying overweight. I see it every day. People at the gym for hours every day and never looking different or moving any better because they are there too long, lack rest, and burn muscle, causing body fat percentages to sway in an unfavorable direction. Not the most ideal way to spend your time and energy. This is not only due to improper exercise and progression, but poor nutrition programming.

Eat real

When I design a nutrition program, I try to stay away from as many processed foods as possible, and try to eliminate wheat all together. I encourage my clients to stay away from it, but if you need to snack on something, go gluten-free. Many times this gets misinterpreted to eat as many gluten-free foods as possible. From pasta to pancakes to corn chips to cereal to brownies, it is still a processed food, and it still needs to be limited, period. Gluten-free foods still have a high glycemic level, still have a lot of empty calories, and can still make you fat. Look what happened in the early 90's fat-free craze. It made people fatter because they removed something and replaced it with something just as bad or worse — fat for sugar, gluten for other processed flours etc. Many of these foods lack nutrients and proteins deeming them useless to the body anyway, so less is better.

In conclusion, there is no magic way to get results. The higher quality food you eat, the better you will feel. The smarter you train, and the more you pay attention and LISTEN to your body, the better you are going to be. Train hard and rest easy!

20

GIRLS (AND GUYS) JUST WANNA HAVE FUN?

D o you just want to have fun?

Who said exercise has to be fun and exciting? Is eating, showering, driving, and brushing your teeth fun and exciting? Do you change these routines to make them more interesting? Do you try handstands while eating to break up the monotony? Do you hop on one leg in the shower so you won't get bored? How about driving to work extra fast and in reverse, just to change things up? I know this sounds incredibly ridiculous, but I see this kind of stuff in the gym every day. People trying to be "new, cool, cutting edge and exciting," with their fitness routines, just to change it up and be more interesting.

It's not fun... It's work

Let's be completely honest with ourselves, exercise isn't very fun. Unless you disguise it with a bicycle, a lake, or a soccer ball, it's a grueling challenge to take the actions to get it done! If it were easy and fun everyone would be doing it, and we wouldn't be in such a physical mess to begin with. It's estimated that only 14 percent of the U.S. population exercises in a regular, effective program. So with this being said, let's accept it for what it is: exercise is work, and it's something that we *need* to do more than *want* to do. It doesn't have to be complicated or fun. You do not need to add variety to every single workout, and you do not need to add variables and tricks to every exercise.

News flash!

Here's a news flash: adding tricks for variety or fun not only looks stupid, it is dangerous. There is no need to do this. Most people are not ready to veer off the path of basic lifts and primal movements such as the squat, lunge, press and dead lift. Saying that, I do like to vary my routines, but a client needs to master certain tasks and moves first. I change sequences, but practice the same movements. If I were to constantly change exercises, mastering them becomes difficult. I see people doing push-ups with their feet elevated when their lower back is so arched it looks painful. In truth, not many people perform basic push-ups correctly anyway, so progressing before you "own" an exercise leads to injury and poor performance. I saw one guy balancing on a stick with a med ball and his feet on a balance board while doing a push-up. Why? There are so many ways to vary the push-up without performing a circus act, why try so hard to be different? Another example, doing jump lunges, using erratic, ballistic movement patterns. What do they do? They set you up for a knee injury, instead of just mastering a normal lunge. I see these silly and dangerous moves all the time in the gym. The other day, a woman was attempting to squat standing on a Bosu platform. When she attempted to do one, her knees bent about 20 degrees while she over-flexed at the waist. She lacked the flexibility to squat on solid ground, let alone on an unstable one. Across the gym, a guy had the same issue, only he put on knee wraps and a belt, loaded the bar with 300 pounds and exercised poor form, instead of lowering the weight and doing it correctly. I realize all these people have good intentions, and everyone who laces up their

sneakers and goes to the gym deserves credit, but I hate to see people setting themselves up for injury, or best case, lack of results and
a waste of time.

(Not) just the basics

My advice to you is to master the basics: the push-up, the pull-up
and the squat. Be able to perform these exercises *perfectly* before you
progress, and add variations. Treat exercise as another necessary
part of your day. Go in and get it done; use the gym as a tool toward
your goal. It doesn't have to be glamorous or dangerous or exciting.
One of my instructors always said, "push something pull something, squat, and do something rotational and you have a routine."
Simple, safe, and effective. When you realize all the good you are
doing for your body — hey — it just might be fun for you, too.

21

FITNESS IS AGELESS — STARTING WITH THE YOUNGEST AMONG US!

I have been asked numerous times by different people about what I specialize in, and I tell them that I don't have a specialty. I like to make everyone better. I have an age range of clients from 14 to 87, and I enjoy training all of them for different reasons.

I also talk to parents and teachers and anyone who will listen about the importance of leading by example, especially for very young preschoolers. If you are going for a walk, take the little ones with you. If you won't eat French fries anymore, then don't order them for your children. When you go out to eat and are careful about ordering healthy gourmet type meals, why opt for mac and cheese or the disgusting chicken finger platter for your children — the ones you love more than life! Remember?

So, first I talk about leading by example. And conversation. Explain what good choices are in food, in what to do with one's time, the importance of outside play over hours of television trances, how you set aside specific time for "workout" whether that is playing a sport, riding a bike, or pulling out the mat and doing your routine right there on the living room floor. Don't shoosh them away. Invite them to watch, or if they can, join in. This establishes lifelong patterns of fitness and healthy eating as a way of life, not something to undo and change (a much harder task).

For those who are a little older, and school is out — wow — what a great opportunity to mold their healthier lifestyles. They will get excited about buying new sneakers, shorts, and swimsuits. They will also get excited about going with you to the market, picking out good food, and making some "let's try this" selections. Add a new food you'll all try together every time you go to the market. If they are going to a day care or sports program or camp, be vigilant about what snacks are fed to your children. If you see neon colored drinks — beware! Don't be afraid to tell the staff what you expect for your child, and what you don't expect. Pack a healthy lunch or provide your own snacks and drinks. Kids need nothing but water to drink — ban the juice!

We know that it's unhealthy

Yes, we know it's unhealthy, and we know it's addictive, yet we still see these items marketed to us. It may have "as much calcium as an 8-ounce glass of milk," but food companies don't trumpet the trans fats, artificial dyes and other nasty stuff in the ingredients.

Here's what is in one popular cheese: *Nonfat Milk, Water, Sugar, Modified Corn Starch, Partially Hydrogenated Soybean Oil, less than 2% of: Cocoa (Processed with Alkali), Salt, Calcium Carbonate, Sodium Stearoyl Lactylate, Natural and Artificial Flavors, Yellow 5, Yellow 6.* That isn't the nutrition you want your kids gobbling, so you should not be including anything like this in their menu.

Once we have a framework down of what we will not feed them, then we discuss what we will include. I ask two questions: Will it make you proud after you've packed it all up that you've done your job by giving them a great lunch and snacks? And the second, important question — will they eat them? I understand the balance between healthy and convenient, flexible and diligent, aware and open. You can pack the world's healthiest lunch, but it does no good if your kids won't eat it. Even if you have to make peanut butter and jelly, purchase the highest quality bread that your child will eat, but without those "no chance" items like high fructose corn syrup or artificial colors. Always get a jelly that's mostly fruit and as natural organic a peanut butter as possible. But even high quality PB&J only takes us so far. To really plan out a menu, before school starts, have a family meeting. Ask your kids what they would like to see in their lunches this year. If you can't get a straight answer, you need to go straight to the grocery store and walk up and down the aisles together. This way you can make informed decisions together, and it won't feel like you are forcing good healthy food on them. Get them excited about fresh fruits, tasty vegetables like carrots, healthy trail mixes, quality breads, and quality deli meats. This will make them happy and you will be satisfied that you are doing a good job as a parent that your kids are really eating healthier.

Playing sports

If they play sports, be concerned about their training. Are they properly warmed up? Stretching? Do they have safety gear? Is injury prevention a priority? If your young ones are starting in competitive sports, make sure they are also strength conditioned — not just learning about great game-winning plays. Strength conditioning will prevent injuries — many that result with sudden stops and starts and pivots. Strengthening the core is vitally important. And don't forget those pre-physicals which can uncover issues that need to be addressed prior to playing sports.

We'll talk more about this next time, but until then, have the best, healthy start to your Summer!

22

Don't be Confused: Metabolic, Strength Training & Cardio

I get the question all the time. *What do I need to do to get in shape?* I always say good nutrition first, but on an exercise level, I advise doing two or three days of strength training, incorporate some functional movements, add some metabolic circuits, and you have a great program to get you strong, fit, and moving better. But, what is metabolic training? What is strength training? What does cardio mean? Run, life cycle, elliptical? What equipment do I need to do this?

<u>Doing something for nothing?</u>

Usually when people in a gym environment say they did cardio, this consists of 30 to 60 minutes of some redundant movement pattern on some motorized piece of equipment lining the walls of the gym, equipped with a TV and magazine racks. You see people lined up, ear buds in their ears, doing the same thing over and over, and getting the same lack of results. This is a waste of time and energy. When the effort doesn't equal results, you are doing something for nothing. The reason behind this is that you get acclimated to the routine, and after a few times, your body no longer responds — it simply has become "used" to doing the routine, rises to the occasion, and results in weight loss / fitness plateaus. When you watch TV, sit down, talk on the phone, or read a magazine while working out, the intensity is non-existent, and the results usually are also.

Metabolic or HIIT training is what it takes to make a difference

The body responds much better to short bursts of intense activity, followed by brief periods of rest, using different movements and routines. This makes the heart and lungs stronger by involving peak contractions, similar to the way you train other muscles. Doing cardio at the same pace only teaches the heart and lungs to be efficient, not stronger. Exercises such as body weight squats, med ball slams, and band rotations can be performed in a sequential order either for time or reps. Followed by rest periods. The rest is important for recovery, allowing you to work out at a higher intensity, therefore netting better results.

Strength training or resistance is the most important type of exercise you can do

When asked, I always recommend strength first. Not only does this make you more stable, but exercises like squats and dead lifts make you move better. Resistance work varies, depending on the clientele. For instance, all my clients dead lift and squat but a 21-year old rugby player uses an Olympic bar weighing 315 pounds, whereas an elderly client lifts a 12-kilo kettle bell. Another big reason to emphasize strength training is that it builds muscle, and muscle is a more efficient tissue at burning calories at rest, allowing us to look better and appear leaner. Building muscle and burning fat are the results of strength training. That's a pretty good return for your investment. Don't do something for nothing!!

23

MISSING THAT HIGH? WHY?

Winter weather is here. And with it, so goes the hanging up of running shoes for a few months. Runners claim there is no better feeling than the runner's high. And they have a hard time adjusting to indoor and treadmill running — they say it's just not the same.

Next time you see a real runner out there on the street — and no question the die-hards will be out there all winter long — look at the expression on their face. Ninety percent of the time I see pain, agony, and misery along with poor form and posture. I study movement patterns all day long by people watching and I notice symptoms such as knock knees, forward head tilt, excessive ankle pronation, supination, etc.

The most problematic issue with today's runners is excessive heel strike. This is due to the excessive padding and elevated cushion heel in today's high tech running shoes. By wearing this type of shoe, you inhibit proprioception (your body's sense of its own position, balance and movement). Seventy percent of that feedback comes from pressure receptions, mostly located in the feet, resulting in reduced sensory feedback and therefore limits the quality of movement and core stability. Due to this and poor posture, 80 percent of runners suffer injuries every year when they practice poor form. On a repetitive basis, you compound dysfunction and probability of injury.

So, my question is, "Why do it when it hurts if most are not very good at it?" And to top it off, the people that are actually good at it with ease of stride and perfect form look thin and frail. Long steady bouts of this type of exercise actually down sizes your heart's capacity making it economize its power so you can go longer. You never push your heart to utilize its reserve capacity, therefore never make it stronger, only more efficient.

Take a winter break

So take a break from all that running and ask yourself, "Where am I going?" Am I really getting more fit? Strengthening my heart? Looking better? Feeling stronger? I suggest running sprints, or doing high intensity interval training. It's more fun, less chance for injury, and you will get in better shape. Look at a sprinter's body if you don't believe me. They are aesthetically much more appealing than most marathoners or excessive runners. I am not telling people that love to run to stop, just follow my philosophy: if it hurts, stop doing it. Read up about running and the new ways we are learning about fitness. Come see me and let's talk. Or better yet, look at some of the people at my gym who look tired, and sweaty, but have a bounce in their step.

24

NO MEDALS
FOR
ALMOST WINNING

"Getting to the gym is half the battle." "Lacing up your sneakers is the toughest part." "At least I am trying." "I eat well most of the time." "I joined, a gym so I took the first step." "I work out when I have time." Are these catchy sayings, or are these just copouts for people justifying their inability to succeed at achieving their fitness goals? If you are reading this, or have been following my column, it means that you care enough about yourself and have good intentions, but good intentions without discipline and follow through will achieve nothing. If you have the desire to strive and be fit, but aren't seeing results, keep reading and you might find out why.

I have a few sayings that may leave a few of you to think I am a little harsh, such as: "You won't get a medal for finishing fourth," referring to Olympians who train hard for years and finish a fraction of a second from the podium. They worked hard and competed, but the reality of it is that effort isn't enough, and you will only get rewarded if you complete your mission. I use this saying for people who tell me they eat well most of the time, but still can't lose the last few pounds because they like to party on the weekends. They tend to get frustrated when I criticize the things they do wrong, instead of giving them credit because they ate a salad on Wednesday! Sorry, I don't make the rules, I just know how to follow them. And the rule is — if you cheat too much with your eating, and drink lots of alcohol, your results will stall, if not regress. When people over 40 say things like, "Hey, I look pretty good for my age," or, "I look better than most people my age," they are just comparing themselves to the masses of people that do less than they do, or look worse than they do, and that is not setting the bar high enough.

Let's face it, statistically only 15 percent of the population care about themselves enough to work out. And the obesity rate is climbing to 30 percent. So what does this tell you about most of the population? If you want to set goals, set them by comparing yourself to people that look like they are 20 years younger than they are, and look at their practices, instead of watching the co-worker who eats donuts and thinking you are better off for eating a muffin. Look at the co-worker who packs her own healthy lunch, or the guy who takes the stairs. Talk to the fittest people around you and ask them what they do for workouts and how they stay in shape. Just don't stay one step ahead of an average sedentary adult, aim higher.

"We strive for perfection, but we will never reach it, because nobody's perfect, but for trying, we will achieve greatness" ~ Vince Lombardi.

I know being perfect is impossible, but I am not a believer in rewarding mediocrity, and words mean nothing unless followed by a course of action. I got frustrated with someone when they told me they were trying to eat better, and when I called them out on the bottle of soda in their kitchen, I was informed that it was diet soda. So, I read the long list of chemicals on the label, but before I finished, an argument erupted as if I was the one who made the soda. This is a person close to me who knows and listens to me preach about food all the time, yet still justifies eating food that causes harm to the body. So, if you know something is not good for you, or has excessive calories, yet you still find ways to justify eating it (it was my friend's birthday), then you are fooling yourself and hindering your progress.

I realize that there is a fine line between telling the reality of things and sounding too critical, but sugar coating (pun intended) things and giving high fives for attempting, talking about, or thinking about doing something isn't going to help someone succeed. In today's world, "almost" isn't going to cut it when you stay up all night attempting to reach a deadline and fail. You will probably lose your job rather than getting a pat on the back for trying, especially if money is lost. Joining the gym isn't going to get you in shape. Yes, it is the first step, but there are many steps you need to take to get and remain healthy. You must decide, and then proceed to make it a lifestyle. You cannot and will not reach a certain level of health and fitness doing it part time. Taking care of yourself requires work, knowledge, and effort, and you need to pay attention to details such as eating quality foods, and meal frequency. In other words, eating at an unhealthy food truck once a day isn't going to do it, even if you work out after. When you see someone who looks great and has lots of positive energy, it isn't because they do things half way. It took desire, drive and discipline. When you want to make a lot of money and be successful, you would surround yourself with like people, and not surround yourself with unsuccessful people. And the same goes for your fitness. Try to surround yourself with fit, like-minded people.

We are all different in many different ways — personality, income, power, intelligence, etc. But a couple of things that make us the same are that we are all given the exact same 24 hours at the beginning of the day, and how you spend it is entirely up to you. Some will waste most of it in front of a TV. Some will let it slide by while sitting in a cubicle. Some will spend it sick in bed. Some will make lots of money. Some will smoke cigarettes, drink and gamble. And some will wake and be productive from the minute their feet hit the floor by doing things that improve their quality of life, benefit their health, and act on the things that will enable them to feel good and be happy. I am a believer that if anyone else can do something, others can also. Nothing is impossible if you invest a little hard work and discipline, and you set goals for yourself. So if you hit a plateau with your fitness, sit back and make an honest assessment of yourself, and try to improve any way you can.

The other common denominator all humans have is an expiration date. Although all are different, very few know when it is, and I am an advocate of quality over quantity. My definition of a quality life is feeling good, infrequently getting sick, moving without pain, and enjoying the things you love to do. These things alone make me want to be fit and healthy and encourage others to do so by spreading the word and educating my audience. It is my nature to have a no-nonsense approach, so if you find me harsh, consider it tough love.

25

TIME IS (NOT)
ON YOUR SIDE

It is something that is infinite, but nobody has enough if it.
It is something that can't be made.
It is something that can't be bought.
It has value, but it is priceless.
It can be spent, but you will never get a refund.

Although it is infinite, we as humans only have a limited amount of it, and nobody will ever know how much they will have. The word of the week is — time. My favorite cliché about time is, "You only have a limited amount, so spend it wisely because there are no refunds." Or, "Life is not a dress rehearsal. There are no retakes." So my question to you is, "Why do you keep wasting it in the gym?"

Yes, I am a big advocate of working out and exercising, but if you are not getting the results you are trying to achieve, then you are wasting your time exercising. I would much rather be hanging out with my nephew, sitting in a coffee shop, reading a book, or lying in the sun somewhere, than being in a gym, accomplishing nothing. Yea, you optimists feel that as long as you get there, that's better than not going, but I am telling you that's the wrong attitude and approach because if you are not exercising properly you are not only wasting your time, but setting yourself up for injury, which is worse.

Efficient — and safe

That's why Fit Body pioneered the 30 minute after burn workout system. We want our clients to get the best results as efficiently and safely as possible. I used to see it every single day: ninety percent of the people in the gym wasting their time and getting nowhere or looking worse. How can this be true you ask? Well this is what I see — people lumbering into the gym (usually with bad posture) grabbing a book or magazine and jumping on an elliptical machine or recumbent bicycle. Then they continue to practice poor form and posture by reading this book or magazine at a pace that would put you to sleep if you watch long enough. You cannot read if you are training intensely, and you cannot train intensely if you are reading. Why bother doing "cardio" if your heart rate isn't going to elevate and you aren't working up a sweat? Sure you may burn a few calories, but if you eliminate a piece of bread or a cookie from your food intake, you have accomplished the same deficit as lollygagging around for 45 minutes. It's not only a waste of time, but by exercising with bad form / posture, you are feeding dysfunction at an accelerated rate which might pay you back with lots of visits to an orthopedic doctor.

My suggestion? Attend three to five of my boot camp sessions a week, grab a partner and go for a fast power walk, or play a game of basketball. Anything to up the intensity, elevate your heart rate, or work up a sweat. On the flip side, you see people killing themselves in the gym, sweating profusely, and slinging heavy weights only to ruin their efforts with a poor nutrition program.

There are two different ways you can sabotage making gains with poor eating:

1) *You eat all the wrong foods.* You finish beating your body down, shredding muscle fibers, and burning up all your muscle glycogen, only to refuel your body with some processed garbage from a drive thru, or some packaged form of protein bar disguised as nutritious

and healthy. Remember your gains are determined by how much rest and how well you nourish yourself AFTER the workout, not how hard you work during it. So if this is your routine, remember you will get fit faster and waste less time if you pay attention to what you eat. Remember, you can't out exercise a bad diet.

2) *Some people do not eat enough.* I'm not sure which is worse. In order to perform at your peak levels in day to day life you need fuel, so when you work out you need even more. When you exercise and lack fuel you end up burning muscle mass which changes your body composition or muscle to fat ratio in an unfavorable way.

I always recommend keeping yourself fueled up and ready to perform at your highest level. If you just want to waste some time, go lay in the grass, and don't waste it in the gym! So if any of this article resonates with you, give me a call and we can get you on the straight line to success.

26

WORK SMARTER, NOT HARDER

Without exercise you won't get fit. Without good nutrition, you won't become healthy.

Many people group the words health and fitness together as if they were synonymous terms. It's hard to believe, but there are vast differences between the two, and I incorporate a system that stresses the importance of both. I will give you an example of how both terms differ, and how to bridge the gap.

Granola guys and gals

The health-conscious people (sometimes referred to as salad eaters, granolas, health nuts, etc.) make sure to only eat organic foods, use non-chemical cleaners, and avoid as many toxic compounds as possible. A wise decision for all. I know someone that even purchased an organic mattress and had the air quality tested in an apartment before making a decision to move in. A little extreme, but health conscious for sure. Many of these people own juicers or, in particular, a Vitamix. Also a smart decision. The biggest mistake this population makes is that they fail to do any kind of strenuous exercise or strength training. Peaceful in nature, the option of walking, gardening, mild yoga, or a cup of green tea and a book is generally more appealing to them than a sweat fest or moving some iron. I believe this is a mistake, because everyone needs to be able to move and lift on a functional level and will at some point need to tackle a set of stairs or chase a child or pet around. And without a solid strength and cardio base, or great movement patterns, daily tasks are difficult or even hazardous, and developing important muscle mass becomes impossible.

Sweat addicted

On the contrary, you have those crazy workout people. You know the ones who kill themselves on the cardio equipment day in and day out to the point of stressing out if they miss a day. Then, they hit a drive thru for breakfast. Or the body builders who go to extremes such as dehydration and steroid use to have that sculpted look. Long distance runners beat their bodies to the point of joint injury and exhaustion, while actually burning up and depleting precious muscle tissue only to become skinny and sick looking. Fitness models, drinking caffeine with artificial sweeteners on the way to the tanning salon, are another example of borderline fanatics. While the majority of these people look like the definition of fitness, they use some unhealthy methods to get that way.

I personally do not believe you need to go to extremes to be both fit and healthy. If you have a temporary goal, such as a body building contest or wedding, OK, but it's TEMPORARY — and not a plan to maintain as a lifestyle. The first step in my system is to build a nutrition program based on whole organic foods. Every member is required to attend a nutrition consultation after they join. I educate them with facts like, if you eat quality foods such as grass-fed beef and lamb, wild caught fish, organic fruits and vegetables, eliminate processed grains and dairy, you are on your way to optimal health. Your body starts to work more efficiently on all levels. Remember, good health is impossible without proper nutrition. We are cellular by nature and every cell is important to nourish so we can achieve ultimate health and build immunity from sickness and disease.

Fitness becomes a lot easier after the first step in my system is applied, because after you incorporate great nutrition, you will only need to work out for three to five 30-minute sessions per week. That's right, we incorporate metabolic and strength training into one high intensity workout that only takes 30 minutes to complete, so you gain muscle, burn maximum fat and you won't over train or beat yourself up for hours at the gym. I tell folks from day one that if health is a priority, then the fitness part will follow. I use the cliché "You can't out exercise a bad diet." Most people just need to step back and use a different approach. Work smarter not harder. And when you incorporate a system like the one we use, it will —
S-ave Y-ou S-ubstantial T-ime E-nergy and M-oney.

27
GET BATTLE READY!

Let's face it, for most of us, life is a bit of a struggle. Unless you are a trust fund baby, or were born with that silver spoon in your mouth, nothing comes easy. Look at self-made millionaires. Most endured years of struggle, late hours, and hard work to get where they are today, and many still put in the hours to maintain their status. Poor people born into unacceptable situations struggle every day. Living in squalor, not knowing where their next meal is coming from, wearing secondhand clothes, well, just isn't a good way to live this life.

Even people in the middle face struggles every day. Supporting a family, paying a mortgage, car payment, private school, or just being able to take a vacation takes days, and weeks of long hours and late nights just to live a middle-class kind of life.

The bad news is that's the way it is at the moment, and there is nothing magical we can do about it except deal with it and conduct our daily lives in the manner in which we *want* to be able to live. Giving up is an option some take, but that will only make matters worse. So, how do we proceed?

Face the fact that nothing worth having will come easy. It's always been that way, and always will be. I believe we are put on this Earth and struggle 'til the day we die, so either fight for survival, or wither away. It's your mentality and mindset that dictates how you will handle the situation, and that's what will dictates your fate.

So why make it worse and live with poor health? I am a Discovery Channel nerd. I love watching programs about the wild, and all the science that shows us how this world was created, and how we have evolved as humans. I was watching a program last week about the rain forest in Brazil, and it dawned on me that every species on this planet faces some kind of struggle. From birth, every species faces a struggle to survive. From birds to lions, either environment or predators make it difficult just to live.

Human beings in the past had the same issues, only we were at a disadvantage. Let's face it, we are not a species meant to physically survive. It was because we are intelligent enough to provide resources and create solutions in order to survive that we still exist.

We don't grow a fur coat in the winter, and we can't withstand long hours in the sun. We don't have protective armor, claws, or venom, we can't camouflage ourselves, nor do we have the ability to out run most animals. Our most vital organs are exposed, and our feet can't withstand the abuse most other mammals can. In general, we are a weak and vulnerable species by nature.

There is good news

But the good news is that we have the intelligence to create fire, shelter, and protective clothing to withstand the elements. We can outsmart predators, and manufacture all the necessities to live a comfortable life. After all, we've been doing it for eons — and we haven't become extinct — yet.

So, my question to you is this…. why are we doing things that ruin our health and make things more difficult for ourselves? Do we not know how lucky we are? Think about it. We have evolved to the point that we don't need to worry about the elements, or some wild animal coming into our dens and eating us. We have resources to live a nice productive life, yet most of us are destroying ourselves by eating garbage food and becoming sedentary. Have we forgotten how lucky we are not to have to look over our shoulders and travel through hell to find our next meal? Why do we choose to live in pain, on medication, be overweight, sick and tired all the time when we have most of the resources — and the intelligence — to take care of ourselves and live a healthy, vital, and productive life?

I hate it when someone says, "I struggle with my weight," or when I see someone unnecessarily living in pain, because I know there are answers so they don't have to do that. They know there are answers, too.

Four things to make your habits

I have a simple formula for ultimate health. It involves four things you must do habitually on a daily basis, and you will be guaranteed good health.

1. Eat clean food. Stay away from packaged / processed garbage and eat only real natural food.

2. Drink enough water. You need to consume half your bodyweight in ounces of water daily to maintain optimal health.

3. Get some sleep. When we sleep, we reset and repair. Lack of sleep is detrimental to your health.

4. Move. Do 30 minutes of exercise daily. (This is why my clients at Providence Fit Body Boot Camp are so fit and strong.)

It's that simple. You don't need to hunt, make clothing, create fire, or struggle to survive. It's all right in front of us, yet the human population is destroying itself by not doing these things.

I didn't write this to be negative, or to depress anyone, but to shine a light on how far we have come, and how far back we are going if most folks don't start making some changes in their life. The struggles will get worse. If you think things are difficult for you now, try doing it in poor health, or doing things in pain and broken down. Realize how fortunate you are, and instead of trying to destroy yourselves, just pay attention, and make some adjustments, and this thing called life that we all struggle with becomes a whole lot better.

Here's the good news. It's not too late to turn it around. The material things that we work for will always come and go, but once our health deteriorates to a certain point, there may be no coming back. If being in top shape and living a healthy lifestyle appeals to you, reach out and seek help from a pro. I am always here for my clients, and if you are not a client already, shoot me a message and I can help you reduce at least one struggle in your life. It's not just about exercise routines with me, it's about helping the "whole you" — diet, motivation, mindset. Once you get "reset," the struggle you may face in other areas of your life will be more manageable — you will be ready for battle. So, let's do it — together.

SECTION THREE

DIET & NUTRITION

1

WANT TO
LOSE WEIGHT?
READY, SET, GO!

There really are only three ways to lose weight. No, it's not as easy as 1-2-3 because it also takes both mental and physical toughness. And you need to set goals. If you are overweight and you follow these three steps, you can expect to lose two to three pounds per week until you reach your ideal body weight. At that point, you will look and feel so much better, it becomes almost effortless to adopt your new healthy habits as a healthy way of living. There is no quick fix, no pills, packaged food, liquid diet, point system, etc. for long-term success, and I don't recommend any of that. What I do recommend is doing what it takes to acquire the desire and discipline to change for the better. Let's assume you have that — and let's review the three steps to reach your goal.

Step 1: Overhaul your nutrition program

We start this by changing the quality of your foods. If you eat potato chips, we change that to organic corn chips. If you eat a commercial yogurt, we swap for an organic / biodynamic farm yogurt with live cultures. We switch out "conventional" vegetables and meats for organic. And the reason is because our bodies work more efficiently when we detox from the elements such as cheap vegetable and canola oils, overly processed dairy, nitrates, corn syrup, soy, wheat, other GMO fillers, and pesticides that cause major inflammation in the body. This step is more important by far than counting calories. Dealing with caloric intake will be the third progression after eliminating certain foods.

Step 2: Get moving

Start slowly and start to move more whenever you are ready. Take the stairs if you are only going a few flights. Park further away from the door. Take some walks at lunchtime or before work. It is important to move to keep the system working properly to help blood flow to extremities, release endorphins, stimulate digestion, release free radicals, and improve sleep, as well as burn calories and feel more energetic. You do not have to join a gym or do anything too strenuous at this point. This is to get the body acclimated to movement. If you do too much, you could get excessively sore or injured which will put a damper on your program and give little incentive to follow through. That's why I believe in progressions. Start small, make attainable goals that you can reach, log your progress, and after a while it will become almost automatic.

Step 3: Progressions on nutrition and movement

Exercise and nutrition are the only ways to lose weight and keep it off, but you have to make adjustments to your program when you reach plateaus. After a while, your body adapts to the changes you make, so we need to make progressions.

Here are some examples of progressions for your eating plan. After you make the quality change, it's time to eliminate more processed foods. Even though it says organic and gluten-free, many of these foods are highly processed and the less you eat the better. Make the transition to whole foods exclusively. The next thing to do when you reach a sticking point is calorie control. Everybody has different requirements and needs, so you need to play with portion sizes. By this point you should have a good understanding of your body's needs, so make some adjustments. Progression in exercise is endless. You go from mild to intense by adding heavier loads and training faster. Go from walking to strength training to super setting to metabolic training to sprinting, etc. This requires some common sense so you do not over do it. The best advice I can give on this is to feel it out and listen to your body, train within your limits, but push yourself. If still confused, hire a professional to stand by your side and encourage you to achieve your goals. There aren't any magic solutions — it's slow and steady that wins the race — but you won't get anywhere unless you start... so, GO!

2

7 STEP PLAN
FOR WEIGHT LOSS

Do you train hard, train regularly, and still can't figure out why your results are minimal? Even non-existent? Here's why. It's not your lack of effort, or the amount of exercise you are doing. It's not the type of training you are doing, unless it's bouts of lethargic, redundant cardio on some machine for an hour. And it's not the intensity of exercise you are doing — it's your nutrition program. Period. Because if you live by a sound nutrition program, all types of exercise will net you results. And if losing weight is the goal, you could do it without ANY EXERCISE. But I am still a big advocate of exercise regardless of anyone's goal, so you didn't hear that from me. But it is true. Master your nutrition and you will be a winner!

Have a plan

Creating a nutrition plan doesn't have to be difficult. You would never know it with the hundreds of books written in the subject, but you can toss all those books away because I am going to give you the "Cliff's Notes" version right now and leave you with an easy map to follow.

1. Remove processed food from your diet, and if you can't totally eliminate all of it, eat gluten-free, and organic options. Wheat, GMOs, sugars, and other various cheap fillers and chemicals are

lurking in commercially processed foods and are sure to derail results and add inches to your waist. And they're also seen as responsible for skin, digestive, neurological, and cognitive problems.

2. <u>Eat fresh fruit and vegetables</u>, and try to eat varieties of both. These foods supply you with valuable nutrients and vitamins responsible for building a strong immune system and cellular repair, and they help to eliminate free radicals in the body that damage cells that cause disease and promote premature aging. I recommend vegetables with every meal, but no more than two servings of fruit daily.

3. <u>Eat breakfast</u>. Eat a healthy one full of protein and unprocessed carbs such as steel cut oats, and raw nuts and granolas. Add eggs and you have a great way to jump start your day and your metabolism.

4. <u>Eat frequently</u>. The best way to stoke a fire is to add wood that combusts easily and burns clean. The same goes for your metabolism. If you throw a big log on the fire, it will smolder and raise a lot of toxic smoke, which is what happens when you only eat one or two big meals a day. They just sit there until you need energy, and what's left gets put into fat storage. I suggest grazing on small healthy snacks like hummus, carrots, apples, peanut butter, almonds, etc., throughout the day to stoke that fire.

5. <u>Stop drinking your calories</u>. Consuming diet drinks, smart waters, sports drinks, most smoothies, and protein drinks, and adding cream and sugar to your tea and coffee adds extra calories or artificial chemicals that you do not need and should avoid. Unless you are juicing organic vegetables, or know exactly what and how many calories you are consuming, *eat* your calories so your body works to digest.

6. <u>Get your fiber and calcium</u> from dark leafy vegetables, grains such as quinoa, brown rice, root vegetables, and forms of raw dairy rather than boxed cereal and highly processed low-fat dairy. Many

people feel they lack these nutrients, so they fall for marketing gimmicks and try to get extra by eating all the wrong things. Stick to the plan and you won't be deficient in these nutrients.

7. <u>Eat quality</u>. It is better to spend a little more and consume quality products when it comes to your health. Shop more frequently and don't buy in bulk. Many times things expire or go bad and the cost ends up averaging out anyway, so put in a little extra work when it comes to nutrition and health. You will achieve your goals faster and feel better doing it!!

3

AH-CHOO!

When summer approaches, we are all chomping at the bit to get outside. Fresh air, warmer temperatures, sunlight, vitamin D, and elevated moods are all wonderful. And then we have pollen and allergies. Not so wonderful. I have heard it many times this week, and it seems like an unavoidable problem to some people. But before you reach for the costly OTC meds, try these simple methods to lessen symptoms.

First, eliminate dairy. Due to the mass production and poor quality of animals from which most of our common dairy products come, as well as heat pasteurization and homogenization, commercial dairy products fall under the category of processed foods. Because all bacteria (good and bad) is destroyed during the "process," dairy products lack the enzymes needed to help our bodies break it down and properly digest it, causing a person to become lactose intolerant. It also causes a histamine or inflammatory effect to the respiratory system. Notice when a kid eats ice cream, their noses start running. That's respiratory inflammation, and not good for sensitive people with allergies.

Wheat products are also better off being avoided due to inflammation caused in the intestinal tract. They cause the villi in the intestines to lay flat, not absorb any nutrients, thus leaving foods intact and undigested causing a condition called leaky gut syndrome. This also comprises your immune system, making it more difficult to combat allergies and fight off foreign invaders.

The infamous "Neti Pot" will help relieve symptoms by flushing the mucus in your nasal cavity. It comes with a saline solution, and you need to use distilled or previously boiled water, at room temperature. You flush one side at a time following the instructions on the box. Feels weird but works great.

Local honey also helps clear some symptoms associated with allergies. Little known fact: the honey should be purchased within a three-mile radius of where you live because the bees need to extract and make honey from the same flowers and plants that are irritating you for the anecdote to work. Your best bet is a local store or farmers market.

There is a compound found in wasabi known as 6-MSITC, which suppresses chemicals that cause nose-closing inflammation, so pile it on and let the drainage begin. Another compound that can subside symptoms is spirulina. Take about 2000 mg a day and inflammation and symptoms should ease. If these remedies don't help you out, you may have to avoid outdoor activity or wear a mask during the worst part of the allergy season. But go ahead and try it because the outdoors is good for you!

4

ARE YOU BEING FOOLISH — OR FIT FOR LIFE?

After an old bodybuilding picture of mine resurfaced last week, I discussed the details of contest preparation to a friend and told him about all the hard work and dedication it took to get there — all the heavy workouts, and the craziest, most restrictive diet you can ever imagine. He asked me if I could do it again. I told him I could, and could do it even better than I did in those days, because I know more and my knowledge has evolved a lot since then. However, I told him I wouldn't because I would have to restructure my whole training concept. Then I started to think of all the changes I have made since then, and all the mistakes I made during those days, and how I was misled into thinking I was a picture of health. Let's rewind 15 years and list what I thought was healthy and the reasons why I was wrong.

I owned a microwave back then, and now I won't eat or consume anything that has been heated or thawed in one. Not even considering of the health issues, I think anything cooked in a microwave tastes horrible. Parts are still cold, while others are scorching hot, and everything tastes like rubber. This is due to the electromagnetic radiation used to provide heat. This also denatures and kills most live nutrients in your food, so you are eating food as nutritious as cardboard, and if you reheat in plastic, this causes the xenoestrogens from the plastic to leach into your food, so now you are eating nutrient deficient food loaded with toxic estrogens. Not a good thing! If you doubt the concerns I raise, just Google "don't use a microwave" and read and watch experts in nutrition and holistic health write about their concerns.

Use the stovetop with stainless cookware. It takes about the same time, or just a little longer than a microwave, and will be better for you.

Here are two other mistakes I was making: eating cheap tuna from a can and using artificial sweeteners. The mentality was to eat high protein, and minimize extra calories. I never thought about the BPA's (chemical that seep in from the can), or the high levels of mercury in the tuna, or the toxic nature of the sweeteners. Now, I do not buy or consume any canned goods, artificial sweeteners, or tuna. Buying fresh foods is more beneficial because the food is live, or has recently been so, and so are the nutrients and enzymes that our bodies need for growth and repair and to keep our immune systems strong. I also only eat wild-caught fish such as salmon, striper, sea bass, halibut, and cod. Larger fish such as tuna, sword, and Mako shark carry a higher concentration of toxins due to their position on the food chain. There appears to be a connection to neurological disorders and problems with cognitive function. So you want to eat the smaller fish. Sardines, mackerel, and anchovies are the healthiest, but are not appealing to everyone's pallet. As far as the sweeteners, not too many people are aware of the health risks, so I won't be repetitive on this topic. To ignore the information that is universally agreed upon ends up being a personal choice — and in my opinion, one which would compromise a good diet moving in the right direction.

Another big mistake I made was buying meat and other food from big discount stores. You know, the ones that sell tires and food in the same store? When you pay discount prices, you get inferior goods. The larger the scale, the lower the quality. Think about it. Can a small organic farmer give the same care to 100 animals as it gives to 1500 animals? Absolutely not. Is the food on a cruise ship with 2500 people on board as good as a small local restaurant that seats 30? Again the answer is no. I have learned over the years that it is rare to find a discount on quality items, from food to tools. Therefore, I only purchase my food from quality markets, and only eat free range and grass-fed meats and poultry. It is better for you, for the small farmer, and for the environment.

I also subscribed to the fat-free craze, eating fruity fat-free yogurt, ice cream, cookies, and baked potato chips. Now I know that anything with a label that states: fat free / no sugar / vitamin enriched / low calorie / high fiber is a bunch of processed over marketed garbage. When you eat something packaged, the less ingredients the better, and if you can't read the label — don't eat it. Fat is better than the cheap fillers and chemicals they put in its place, and fat lowers the glycemic index on foods, making them more sustainable and available to be broken down in the body as nutrients. So, when they process yogurt by removing the fat, and add fruit with high fructose corn syrup, it makes it a high glycemic food making the consumer fatter and fatter and more and more insulin resistant, and closer to obesity, and diabetes. Not an ideal place for you to be. Eat snacks with ingredients you can read like: peanuts / dates and salt or potatoes / salt / oil (real organic chips). Less is better, and you will see and feel the difference.

Back then, obesity and other diseases were less than half as prevalent as they are today. I made these changes as soon as I knew the difference, and here I am 15 years later, healthier and fitter with more endurance than I have ever had, with my blood labs and hair analysis tests all being ideal, which leads me to believe that I am correct on these matters. Remember people, knowledge is power, and it took a lot of education and research. Now I am giving it to you first hand in concentrated form. It is up to you to make the change. I changed, and I was enough of an authority then that people asked me for advice. I still knew more than most, but not enough. You now know enough to make a change. If you care about yourself you will make it. Ignorance is no longer an excuse.

My definition of insanity: when you keep doing something over and over, expecting a certain response, and the results never change in a positive way, but keep getting worse. Stop the insanity, and live!!

5

ARE YOU SKINNY FAT?

If you are a woman size four and your arms and legs jiggle because your skin is hanging off the bone, you are *Skinny-Fat*. Here are some reasons why this is the case:

* You do too much cardio

* You do not get enough rest

* You do not do strength training

* You starve yourself / cut calories

To give you a simplified solution:

1. Lay off cardio & let your body heal. Stop wasting the valuable nutrients your body needs to gain muscle.
2. Strength training and building muscle will make you tone and fit and aesthetically more appealing.
3. Eat the proper amount of nutrients. You cannot build muscle without the proper raw materials.
4. Rest. Your body cannot utilize nutrients and repair damaged cells without sleep.
5. Drink quality water and hydrate your body.

Attention! It's an epidemic!

This country is facing an obesity epidemic. Around one third of the U.S. population is now considered to be obese. Along with obesity comes a whole chain of reactive ailments such as diabetes, heart disease, arthritis, and psychological problems like depression these lead to the over use of prescription medication and a broken health care system. So why is this happening? Do we not know? Who is responsible? Who do we hold accountable?

Let's blame companies

Yes, that's the easy thing to do — let's blame the companies that make toxic dyes and chemically made colors that go into most breakfast cereals and bottled drinks, or the marketing companies that do test after test and figure out ways to get kids addicted to these foods and drinks. Then there are the makers of Ritalin who have a cure for the ADHD and neurological damage caused by above such chemicals, and then there are doctors too eager to pre-scribe meds, rather than preach healthy lifestyle habits such as balanced nutrition and exercise. Or we could blame the makers of all these cheap vegetable oils that are in 90 percent of all commercially manufactured food. This is the stuff high in omega 6 fatty acids, the stuff responsible for high LDL (bad) cholesterol. Then we can blame the industrial farmers who are mistreating and raising animals in inhumane conditions, feeding them garbage and other forms of cheap corn and soy based feed to fatten them up faster. How about the government? Should they be accountable for our health? They are the ones, after all, who allow these things to happen legally. They allow the lobbyists to get laws vetoed that would inform the public about what's in products. They let this stuff enter our food supply, turning a blind eye to these mega industrial food manufac-turers, all for profits and bottom lines. So who is accountable?

Look in the mirror

That's right, it's you. We all need to be accountable for our own health. No one else can do it for us. Supermarkets are lined with colorful products full of sugar that addicts us. Fast food is on every corner, electronic devices exist to keep us indoors — it's an endless battle and only the strong and determined will survive. The stuff is out there, and it is your responsibility to avoid it. Just because a vehicle is capable of speeds of 160 mph, doesn't mean the manufacturer is accountable if you crash at this speed? No, it is up to you to take responsibility. I ask if there weren't any health insurance, and you had to pay the doctor yourself, would you still abuse your body? Chances are you wouldn't. So let's not blame big food or big pharma, fast food chains, or the Big Gulp. Don't blame the government, or canola oil. No need to attend a ban Monsanto rally, just be accountable for your own health, take care of yourself by eating quality organic whole food, get plenty of exercise, and eventually all the bad stuff won't be able to survive. If you don't know how, or can't do it alone, hire a coach. The odds are against us, but the underdog never quits.

Good health is attainable, but nobody can do it for you. Take accountability and live well!

6

CALORIES —
IT ALL ADDS UP

"I went out for dinner last night, and wasn't that bad with my eating." I hear this all the time and I am sure many other trainers have heard some variation of this story. I wrote an article a few weeks ago about the cost of being healthy and how you can be on a budget, yet still do it. But let's face it — most training clients are not on a very tight budget. And one would think things are easier when you can afford trainers, cooks, massages, and high-quality food. But the problematic flip side to this is that this type of person eats out more frequently and attends more social gatherings and business events all which center around social eating.

So, I am going to give you a few examples of where your calories are coming from and why you won't make any improvements eating out. First, you sit down and order a drink. Let's say a glass of wine. OK, so let's start adding. That's 80 calories of sugar on an empty stomach. Great way to get the insulin in your system out of control! Because you do not want to get tipsy, you reach for the bread, but you are health conscious, so you opt out of the butter for the healthier olive oil, which still carries 120 calories per tablespoon that is easily absorbed into the bread. Then add 40 calories just for the bread itself. So, with a conservative figure of one glass of wine and one piece of bread with oil that equals 240 calories before you touch a morsel of "real food." And I say conservative because after the first drink, inhibitions get weak, and spiked blood sugar causes excessive hunger, so eating just one piece of bread or having one drink is unusual.

When multiple couples dine, often appetizers are ordered family style. Unless everyone is health conscious, there is a good chance some pizza or fried calamari will be included. But you order a salad, "with dressing on the side, please." Guess what! Figure another 120 calories worth of oil / dressing, some blue cheese crumbles and the salad, plus just one bite of something — a taste even — and that brings the appetizer round to a modest 200, and 440 total calories going into the dinner round.

Now we are primed and ready to eat, but trying to be fit requires sacrifices, so you shoot for the healthy omega 3's and order the salmon with quinoa and vegetables. As healthy as it is, we still need to add 157 calories per 4-ounce piece of fish which is about half an order in most places, and quinoa carries 170 calories per half cup, and cooks are more concerned about taste than calories so the olive oil runs rapidly in the kitchen adding hundreds of calories to a meal. So, let's figure 450 calories on dinner plus the previous 440, and now we have 990 calories if we pass on dessert. And many people eat out more than once a week. That is half of a lot of people's daily requirements on one meal.

Now don't get me wrong, I am not a big calorie counter, and I advise people to up the quality of their food first, and in most cases, they lose weight and will feel less bloated / inflamed eating quality food. I won't start counting calories until results hit a plateau, but I always recommend grazing and spreading them out among five to six feedings, not one or two. When you consume this many calories in one sitting, you will gain weight. Guaranteed. And the example I just detailed is someone ordering with some concept of healthy food. THIS IS A MODEST ESTIMATE of a meal in any restaurant. I want to make it clear that I am not bashing restaurants, or trying to deter you from eating out and being social, because there are many good ones. I am just trying to create awareness as to where your calories are hiding, and remind you to pay attention to small details to live healthier. So go out and enjoy food, just don't kid yourself about the number of calories you are eating. And stop scratching your head and guessing why you are not reaching your goals.

7

CONVENIENCE IS
A RISKY THING

onveniences: do they hurt more than they help? I figured out a
way to help solve this nation's obesity epidemic. Are you ready
for this? Stop producing automobiles that have a functioning
driver's side window. How is this going to help? Because it makes the
concept of the drive-thru window obsolete. We will actually have to get
out of our car and go into a restaurant to eat, and these places that sell
fast garbage foods won't be such a convenience. We have become such
a nation of laziness and inactivity, that these places capitalize on the fact
that we so often look for the easy way out. I am all about efficiency, and
convenience, and finding the fastest way to do something, but not when
it puts our health and well-being at risk which is what most "convenient" options do.

Drive-throughs. Keep driving

Let me give you some examples, and hopefully you'll think twice before
opting for the easy way. Fast food restaurants. Yes, they are easier and
faster, but a majority of them sell nothing but processed, commissary
produced garbage foods, shipped frozen in boxes and plastic contain-
ers. They shouldn't be sold for human consumption. Burger places generally sell frozen industrial farmed raised beef loaded with byproducts
and fillers. They hire our teenagers to work in assembly lines and as-
semble your pre-made food from compartments in a make unit. Cheap

and fast. Until it all ends up stored around your waist. Then it becomes a long and cumbersome chore to burn it off.

If it's chicken you are in the mood for, and you have been disillusioned into thinking that it will be healthier, I have bad news for you. It's not. In fact, the biggest fast food chicken chain doesn't even use the word chicken in its name anymore because it isn't really chicken. They, too, raise animals on unsustainable farms, and load their "chicken" products with byproducts and fillers, and produce it in bulk to cut costs so you can buy it cheap and fast. Yum, right? Even the rotisserie chicken you buy from fast food places is loaded with coloring and nitrates, and the side dishes aren't any better because they are loaded with butter and cooked in cheap GMO canola oils. Yes, it's true, you can go grab lunch for under $10, and in about four minutes, but what does it cost in the long run?

Convenience stores

I run out of coffee on occasion, and need to stop at a convenience store for my morning fix. And with the exception of a basket of bananas, there isn't anything really edible in the entire store. I cringe when I see school kids come in before class and load up on colorful processed chemical poison in a wrapper, or the construction workers who grab some sort of "breakfast" sandwich in a plastic package and then toss it into the microwave. Little do they know that the food alone is causing harm to their bodies. And when you microwave items in plastic, toxins transfer right into your food, so you are not only eating processed garbage food, but getting a large dose of xenoestrogens — a neurotoxin in the body that causes cancer and harms the neurological system. Even the yogurt and granola bars they disguise as healthy will put unwanted inches on your waistline. Again, not very convenient when you save ten minutes but cost yourself countless hours in the gym to undo the damage.

Technology

The last "convenient" thing I want to talk about has nothing to do with food, but has a lot to do with some of the social and economic demise of this great country, and that is — technology. Yes, it has its place, and can make our lives easier and more efficient. We can even save lives with the amazing new medical technologies. But, like many good things, we can abuse it.

I do believe we have come to that point where our technologies are causing physical and social dysfunction to society. They have an impact on an economic level. Tech companies do employ people with skills in the field, but go to a bookstore today (if you can find one) where you can actually touch the pages and read. The results that come from lack of a reading society are obvious. But, there is also the commerce that came from the book industry — empty real estate in strip malls and larger shopping centers, real estate that sits empty and people losing income along with those who have lost their jobs. In addition to the simplicity of ordering books or reading books online, there has been a bigger effect than meets the eye. And, it's having a ripple effect. Look what it's done to us, physically. Bad posture from having our heads down looking at a device, or sitting all day, inactive children who used to play outside, but now choose video games as an option for entertainment. We used to have to get up and go somewhere, have human interaction with someone, and physically exert some effort to purchase products. But now, everything is on a screen at our fingertips, and as a nation, we are paying a steep price for it.

Cost of all this convenience

We all need conveniences in our lives. We all get busy and like to simplify certain things, but we need to stop and start analyzing what it is costing us in the long run and decide if most of these things are conveniences or a quicker means to a sad end. Dishwashers are a great thing, trash compactors even better. But driving up to a window for your food isn't. Step back and figure out what's more important to you, saving five minutes now might be just costing you and your family your health and vitality later.

8

COST-FREE WAYS TO GET HEALTHIER

Stop drinking calories
Stop buying in bulk
Stop serving family style
Move a little more

Unless you are juicing 100 percent organic vegetables, I do not advise you to drink your calories.

That is, unless you want to gain weight. Even juicing people get carried away and add too much fruit and calories to their juicing and smoothies. Juicing is a great way to get concentrated nutrients into your system, but it is easy to consume too many calories at one time. I see it daily at the gym. People workout, then hit the smoothie bar and purchase a protein drink loaded with artificial sweeteners, sugars, and all sorts of "add-ins." I see graham crackers and Oreo's as options. C'mon man… although consuming high calories and simple carbs after an intense workout is beneficial, and absorbed into muscles more rapidly, due to low glycogen stores, I believe quality carbs such as sweet potatoes and brown rice or quinoa are better choices for sustained energy. Even sport drinks and low calorie "diet" drinks cause setbacks when you are seeking optimal health and performance. Stick with pure clean water, and you will save lots of money and calories. By the way… coffee has minimal calories, until you add cream and sugar, so keep that in mind.

282

Stop buying in bulk

Just stop it. Go back to times when we put thought into our meals and stopped at the market a few times a week — a bag at a time. That way you aren't loading up on things that tempt you. Even if you want them, tell yourself, "oh, I'll buy them the next time I come in" — and then don't. Try doing this and I think you'll find that in total, you will spend less, eat healthier, and get some exercise, too. I find that marketing (stopping at a fresh air market, roadside stand or specialty store) also helps transition from work to home. It's good for your mood and mental health.

Eat with your family, but don't eat "family style"

It is very difficult for anyone NOT to overeat when there are large bowls of food on the table in front of them, especially if the food is delicious. It is very easy to grab an extra spoonful of potatoes, rice, meat, etc. if it is within reach… and wham! An extra 150 calories that you didn't need or want, and you just ate it because it was available. Instead, always plate the food in the kitchen, and leave the remainder in pans on the stove. Fill half the plate with vegetables, a quarter with wheat-free grain, a quarter with your protein, and serve. Save the leftovers for a healthy lunch tomorrow. Or you could serve buffet style. Try being the server for your family as they come up to the counter so you can control portions, especially for children who may have eyes bigger than their stomachs — or bigger than their stomachs should be eating.

Move a little more

It's always free and always beneficial. Let's face it folks, it gets really easy to be inactive with all the luxuries we provide ourselves. We sleep, hopefully for eight hours, then sit for breakfast, sit on the way to school or work, sit at work, sit for lunch, sit for dinner, sit and watch TV, then the cycle repeats itself. I say break the cycle. Wake up and do some stretches / push-ups, then park a little further away from the door instead of waiting for the front spot. Take the stairs. Stand up and stretch every hour. Get on a program and make movement a priority in your day. It stimulates circulation, stretches tight muscles, strengthens weaker ones, and gets you out of a seated slumped over position, saving your posture. Now get up — do it now — and move!

9

DON'T BE A TURKEY

The holidays — take Thanksgiving, as the most perfect example. You say, it's OK, I am going to stick to my guns. I am making and bringing my family a Brussels sprout platter and a sugar-free dessert. I won't have mashed potatoes or stuffing. I am not going to eat badly on that day. Right?

H
a!I bet I had you going now, didn't I? You're thinking that because I am a trainer this would be true, but everything I just wrote is really just one big lie. Because I am going to cheat and enjoy doing it — and you should also. It doesn't make sense to stress yourself out and ruin your day. You are spending time with family and should enjoy it. What? You think that a personal trainer who always preaches eating healthy is telling you to go ahead and cheat? Yes! That's right. Because you are lying to yourself if you think you can make it through a holiday with such delicious food at hand — like my favorite homemade apple pie — and not cheat. I am not going to fight homemade pecan pie, homemade sweet potato casserole, or any other delicious dessert item I may encounter. I am going to enjoy this day and not be concerned about over indulging. But, as with most good things, they come to an end. So, by the end of the day, it will. And here are some tips to get you through that day, without totally losing it, and find your way back on track the next day.

Turkey time

At dinnertime, fill your plate with vegetables and turkey first, then add the sweet starchy carbs after. You will eat fewer calories and still enjoy the heavy stuff. After dinner, wait a few minutes before having dessert. Stand up and stretch out, or maybe go for a walk. Watch some football. Then for dessert, have small pieces and just sample the spread. Don't take home leftovers or extra dessert. Do not let this binge carry over until Monday. If you take leftovers home, take the healthy stuff like vegetables and turkey and not those desserts that will sit on your counter, and remain in your presence, after Thursday.

The "day after" workout!

Lift some weights. Go to Providence Fit Body Boot Camp, or a Fit Body Boot Camp in your area, for a fat burning muscle-building workout. Your muscles will feed off the glycogen from all the carbs and sugar you ate. You may get the best workout you've ever had. Whatever you do, do not let yourself fall into a rut. Do not throw your arms in the air and say I'll let the weekend go and start again on Monday. You must get back on track the very next day.

Have a plan

Remember how long it took to get results, and how important that's been to you? So be careful you do not throw those results away in just a few days. Let's be realistic folks, you may try, but it is unlikely to stay on your nutrition plan for the holidays. But you can control the damage and keep weight gain to a minimum. You do that by getting back on track and continuing your routine. Work out on Thursday, if you can, but definitely on Friday. At least you will burn a lot of the calories you consumed. Remember Friday is a weekday, but many people have it off — but do not consider it an extension of Thursday. Thanksgiving is a one-day holiday. So, when it's over, resume eating like you do on your weekly routine, and maintain your healthy habits.

I hope these tips will help you and keep you from sabotaging your progress. Enjoy the day, everyone — be thankful for family and friends. And for your health!

10

EASY TO BE MISLED

Many think that if their diets aren't up to par, they can just exercise a little harder and it will make up for it. If you think exercising without eating properly is enough, particularly for weight loss, it's not. I currently have two clients who train with me, and they work very hard during our sessions — very little rest, high intensity workouts — and they come always motivated to do the program. But the weight they hoped to lose while getting more fit, is very slowly coming off. The reason is that they do not pay close attention to their eating and drinking program. I do "preach" to them almost every time we work out, but one is a gourmet cook who frequently entertains, and is also a fine wine aficionado, so my recommendations and advice goes somewhat unheard or gets sidelined. Recently, this client's friend lost 20 pounds without thinking very much about intense exercise. All through diet! Suddenly we have a change of heart happening — and a supermarket tour and shopping trip is on the calendar. I know that a few tweaks to eating habits, and shopping at healthier markets and farmer's markets, will restore the path to total health and weight loss at a much faster pace. So if you think exercise is enough, you could be expending time and effort for minimal results. You won't make up for a weekend of rich foods and alcohol by running into the gym on Monday morning. If you want to get the most out of the time you spend exercising, you need to eat, rest, and recover properly!

The "other white meat"

Pork has been called the "other white meat." Why? Because it is lower in fat, or carries a label that says it is "low sodium" or "nitrate free." Pork products, of course, come from pigs. Most pigs have been raised in inhumane conditions, are still fed what we consider garbage, along with antibiotics. The outcry and call for humane conditions that we see around cows and chickens hasn't really included pork. As Jules said in Pulp Fiction "Pigs are filthy animals." This holds true on the inside, too. A pig has a shorter digestive system than a cow does, so food and digestive enzymes are eliminated too fast for ultimate filtration, leaving bacteria and toxins behind to accumulate in the meat. If you really need to eat pork products, it is essential you purchase only certified organic pork products, just as you should with chicken and beef.

Buy local!

Just because something is local doesn't make it good for you. Whenever I visit a farmer's market or roadside stand, I always ask if it is organic, and most of the time the response is, "no, but we're local." Well, local pesticides are just as harmful as those used in other states. Washing the exterior of the product helps, but doesn't eliminate toxins absorbed into the soil and root system. So the question you should be asking is, is the corn organic? Is it GMO free? If the answer is no, now the choice will be yours. Most local animals are raised humanely in pastures, so eggs, chicken, and beef are good products. Just ask if it is free range and/or 100 percent grass fed.

I believe in supporting local merchants and farmers as long as they are up to quality standards, disclose the information, and they price their goods to be affordable. The issue of supporting big label products that come here from other countries, bypass local distributors, and sell at the same or high price is a big issue for me. So, I ask questions, I make educated decisions, and most of all I don't assume anything. You may want to do the same. Remember — don't assume "local" means "organic." Being an informed consumer makes you smarter in selecting your foods, and it also will serve to encourage the vendors to listen to what consumers want. That is how we have developed local farmers' markets, organic foods, and more. Your voice is powerful — so are your questions!

11

EAT THIS, NOT THAT

Let's talk about the food we eat. So much of this is in the news every day! Eat this, not that. The information is confusing, and people just don't know what to eat, and what to buy. While not getting into breaking down macro nutrients and counting calories, I do want to give you a basic understanding of what foods I recommend you should be eating as well as what foods you shouldn't — and why.

Factory foods

Due to large food manufacturers spending millions of dollars marketing their products, and trying to deceive the public, eating healthy has become more difficult than ever. Even when you know what to eat, it can be difficult to find the proper foods in traditional supermarkets and in restaurants. When I hear the word "factory," the first thing I envision is a large or complex with pipes taking chemicals "in," and tall stacks taking wastes and pollutants out. Inside are teams of people working in protective gear, hazmat suits and gas masks. And, yes, it is very much like that in large food factories. Now ask yourself if you want a place like this making your food? The sad truth is that most Americans eat food that comes from this type of manufacturing setting. So this is where we can begin: STOP EATING FOOD MADE IN A FACTORY! This includes processed foods and grains as well as animal products that have been mass-produced. Ask yourself if the animals were raised with care and pride, or were they treated like some other commodity, such as plastic or Styrofoam?

GMOs

Today, just about anything containing soy, wheat, and corn has been produced in an outdoor manufactured way, with large cash crops being turned into GMOs (genetically modified organisms). There are too many reasons NOT to consume GMOs for me to list, but if you Google dangers of GMOs, you will find a plethora of good, detailed information. For the purpose of overall health, our bodies do not break down, digest, and utilize these foods efficiently, which causes great stress and inflammation to the body. So when we eat something that doesn't get broken down and is used as energy or building blocks for muscle, it gets stored as fat.

Farms

Another thing to be wary of is the way your animal sources are produced. Larger "feedlot" farms are notorious for mistreating animals, keeping them in confined areas, and feeding them all sorts of processed, garbage foods that fatten them up quickly. When you feed animals huge amounts of processed grains they get fatter faster. Is there a relationship to humans gaining weight and being heavier than ever? Avoid eating this stuff. Look for grass fed beef, lamb, bison, free range chicken, eggs, and pork, and consume only wild caught fish. If you don't carefully select your animal sources, you are eating all the toxins and antibiotic drugs they consumed, magnified! Fat in their bodies as well as ours store toxins, so the more of these inferior products we consume, the more toxic matter we consume, and the sicker we get. Animals that are allowed to roam, forage, and eat what they were biologically designed to eat (cows / grass, chickens / seeds and insects, etc.) provide us with more nutrients, vitamins, minerals, and amino acids that our bodies need to maintain a strong immune system, build muscle, burn fat, and be healthier, energetic, more vital and efficient. You will also be supporting farmers who treat their animals in a humane fashion and a much more sustainable closed organic cycle.

Organic and local

The last important thing to consider is whether your produce was grown organically or conventionally. Some argue that the difference in nutrients is minimal, so consider other factors. Conventional growers use pesticides that can not only harm workers spraying them (hence the gas masks they wear), but also kill all the micro-organisms needed to replenish the soil in a closed organic cycle. Sure you can wash your produce and peel the skin, but what about the chemicals that are absorbed through the soil? These compounds are widely believed to cause conditions related to the central nervous system, as well as neurological disorders, infertility, ADHD and behavioral issues, etc. So, you may be willing to chance it, but I recommend you begin transitioning to eating organic produce, or at least local, where you know it was picked fresh and seasonal. Conventional mega-farm growers grow in mass quantity pick prematurely, spray with gases to slow ripening, and wait for the prices to sway in their favor — not the practice I want to support.

This is just the tip of the iceberg when being nutrition-conscious, but the most important things to remember are: avoid highly processed foods, eat only humanely, sustainable raised animal products, and eat organic and local as much as possible. By doing this, you will eliminate many factors that can slow your goals to achieving a healthy fit body, as well as many ailments such as inflammation and arthritis, and many sicknesses and diseases.

While this all may appear daunting and difficult, don't be discouraged. Take the challenge to learn more about the foods you eat, both for you, and your family. Visit the local farmer's markets, stop at roadside stands this summer, plant a garden, find local organic farms, buy your seafood off the docks, ask questions... Yes, there will be an increase in your food budget, but the more consumers demand better foods, the more businesses will hear what we want and adapt their products. Just think about all the restaurants now that offer gluten free menus. Consumers have power, so let's use our voice and also let our dollars speak for us as we patronize businesses who listen.

12

FRIENDS?
LET THEM EAT CAKE.

We talk a lot about eating right and working out in ways that will get you results. You want to join the right gym and make sure you are eating good, wholesome foods and not junk diet foods. Get rid of those sugar-laden beverages and opt for clean water. But what can often derail you from your best laid plans are those who are closest to you — your family, friends, co-workers and acquaintances. Today, I want to talk about these people and how important their support can be to your success.

Common sense

It's common sense to know that you want people around you who will support you when you start any new venture — whether it's a new job, a marriage, having children, or changing your life around to be healthier. You assume everyone around you will be pulling for you. They'll encourage you to bring out your best, right? Change your schedule to include gym time. Change your menu at home. Change what you eat — and drink — when you go out. Change the way you dress. Even the way you talk or how your thought processes have turned from negative to positive. You're pushing up against and resisting laziness, temptation, and negative thought in yourself. You come to the gym not only for guidance and skill, but for being around those who will support you, too.

Be strong against those working against you

As a fitness professional, I have seen many clients who want to turn their lives around by adopting new healthy fitness regimes. And I've heard their stories about the negativity around them, too. People, for whatever reason, may not want you to succeed, including friends who are as overweight as you, or those who are lucky to have a metabolism to be naturally slim and fit looking. They are the ones who will encourage you to have those fries as a side at the restaurant, or buy one more drink. Or, your family members, though they love you, might not like this new healthy way you have of cooking, or might tempt you with cookies and cake. They might even think what many people have commented about me, that this lifestyle is too strict, overboard, and even neurotic. They just don't see what we do. They don't see this passion we have for life, for taking care of ourselves, for feeling good about who we are and what we have accomplished.

Like you, when I am out socially or with family, and someone says, "Eat this dessert (usually some chemical laden fake food from a supermarket chain), you need to live a little," it drives me crazy. I go out of my way and encourage others to have the knowledge and discipline to avoid these foods, so how is this living it up? Eating something that is going to make me tired, feel lousy, maybe feed disease, and sabotage the time I spent working out, is not living it up in my book. But eating a nice filet medium rare or getting a good night's sleep, is!

Fight the resistance

When you are out with friends, and you stay out later than you wanted to, or you drink too much maybe due to peer pressure, or you get the "C'mon let's have one more" or "I don't like to drink alone" or "Just one shot for old times." Remember: you are the one that has to suffer the next day. You will be dehydrated, tired, have a headache, or feel nauseous — you will be useless and miserable because you didn't show enough discipline. It's your choice; but I suggest you fight against this pressure.

You know what's right

Don't we tell people to avoid something bad even if everyone else is doing it? We tell that to our kids, and we were raised with that advice. So, let's not give in to peer or society pressure, and let's make the right choices. It's all about you doing it for yourself, because no one else is going to do it for you. Big food manufacturers don't want you to eat healthy food; there's no profit for them. Even healthcare settings are said to be more about managing illness than keeping you healthy.

Let them join you

One way to fight against that constant temptation and what I call "resistance" is to let those around you just watch you as you reach your goals — as you feel better, look better, and become a more positive a friend to have around. Make no mistake, fighting this fight to be healthy is all out war. And you need to fight it, because you've decided you want to. So, turn a deaf ear to those who tempt and doubt you. Read inspiring information and blogs, then follow us on social media. Come, hang out in the gym, and watch people just like you sweat and delight in their success. There's a high five here for you — even if there isn't one for you at home or when you're out with friends. Maybe not yet. But, here, you can count on it.

13

OBESITY:
WHY HEALTHY EATING
AND EXERCISE
CAN SOLVE
THE PROBLEM

W**hen you treat obesity like a disease,** the burden on the healthcare system will grow, and it does nothing to fix this problem at its roots. I get this odd mental picture of someone standing under a bridge with a life preserver instead of installing a curb and a guardrail before there is a crisis. We do need to address the root cause of the obesity problem, and it starts with awareness, education and prevention. Once someone is obese, and their blood sugars are abnormally high, their respiratory systems are not functioning properly, and every movement is a struggle. One's will power, discipline, desire, and sense of self-worth diminishes making it more difficult to stick with any health program. Preventing weight gain from getting to this point should be our goal, particularly as we age.

How we avoid getting to this point is by educating people about how to eat and exercise, of course, but also by starting from the top down. The government needs to pay more attention to nutrition and exercise, beginning with programs in schools and then providing incentives to employers to promote health and wellness in the workplace. Helping the organic / biodynamic farmers so healthy eating becomes affordable and accessible to everyone, not just the few, is another top down program that will help, as well as not giving subsidies and tax breaks to large industrial farms and food manufacturers that are responsible for our crisis to begin with. These efforts could do so much to address the ballooning of our bodies — and the ballooning of our healthcare costs.

The role of inflammation in the body

Another big problem people face and one that can cause a chain reaction of effects on the human body is inflammation. Whether it be sore joints or an upset stomach, or skin conditions, people are buying anti-inflammatory drugs in record numbers, causing a whole new group of underlying problems and side effects. Let's remember Vioxx for a moment, and the rush to make this a miracle drug that caused serious problems for so many people. Before that it was the magic weight loss medication, Fen Phen. In the rush for a silver bullet, the side effect was to destroy people's heart valves causing irreparable harm, and it was taken off the market with litigation still going on today. Let's hold off on those drugs, and once again get to the root of the problem.

What are the causes of inflammation in the body? Some are food allergies, poor diet with lots of processed food, wheat and dairy, unbalanced hormones, or chemicals. Most cases of inflammation can be alleviated by just cutting wheat and dairy from your diet and doing some basic movement. How could changing our diets dramatically impact inflammation? The reason this happens is that the food industry has denatured these foods to the point where your body treats them like foreign invaders instead of useable nutrients, and your digestive tract goes into a fight or flight response, just like your immune system fighting a disease. Hence, fever and inflammation. Notice when you eat certain Chinese food you can't get your ring off and your watch is tight? Or your feet swell in your shoes and your ankles look puffy? That's inflammation. And it's another place we can start to put our own good sense into our diet and reduce the damage being caused to our body.

Another area is prescription medications

We just shake our heads when the television commercial for some drug has 10 seconds of good things it might do for us, and 20 seconds of adverse side effects. Really listen to those side effects. They are there because the government says they must be there, because science has shown that these things can happen to you, and that you need to be risk informed. Before you begin taking medications like this, again, stand back and reassess the situation. If the side effects of a drug to help you quit smoking sound worse than if you just smoked, well, I'm almost inclined to say keep smoking because at least we know more about the damage we're causing. But of course, for most of us, we need to do the hard work to make it happen — go to smoking cessation programs, find what works for you, get disciplined about it, and you can succeed.

I'm not telling you not to listen to your doctor and not to take a medication. Not at all. What I am saying is stop looking first for a magic pill or a magic cure. We're conditioned to do that. Begin with a simple philosophy — "first, do no harm." Then really learn what you can do about being overweight, or too sedentary, or how to quit smoking or drink less. Make a few simple adjustments to your lifestyle — when you have success at them — make some more. Do what you can to dedicate yourself to health and wellness, prevention and a natural lifestyle. Again, I'm not saying to avoid medical care, not at all, and I don't believe that you can cure every condition and illness with nutrition and exercise, but I believe you can prevent many of our chronic diseases from setting up in the body this way. I truly do.

If you adopt a healthy program before health issues start or before weight gain gets out of hand, you can go a long way to staying out of the medical system. You will be healthier. Once you are sick, and once you are on high treatment regimes, it is difficult to get out of them. It seems that one medication always leads to another. One disease brings on another and requires more medical care. Just think if we could catch a weight problem before it became obesity, or before it became arthritis, hypertension, diabetes or cardiovascular disease.

Our medical costs are rising

They are rising for us as individuals more so than ever before. The system has reached a critical mass. We do have power against this — we have knowledge and people to help us. In addition to obesity and all the complications it can cause, we can impact allergies, sexual dysfunction, asthma, depression, back and orthopedic problems, and the list goes on and on. As we watch the healthcare system gear up to change, there are many questions we won't have answers to about how this will work, until we get there. But we do know the steps we can take — now. We can go for a walk, start a regular exercise program, eat some kale and green leafy vegetables with turmeric, whole eggs, cinnamon, or something that nature produced.

Take a step back

We can read more about nutrition and become self-educated. We know that to go forward, sometimes we must all take a step back. Learn how we were meant to eat, and how we were meant to move, to sleep, to rest, and rededicate ourselves to that. Do it not only for ourselves, but for our children and our families so we can go forward healthier than we have been, smarter than the food companies, and more in control of own health costs and destiny.

14

IT SAYS IT'S HEALTHY RIGHT ON THE LABEL! RIGHT?

I have dealt with many people who claim they can't get the results they want no matter how hard they try. The first thing I ask them is about their eating habits. Nine out of ten times, people tell me that they eat "pretty well." They are not telling me this because they are trying to lie to me, but due to false marketing and media claims, they are disillusioned into thinking they are eating healthy. That is until I have them do a detailed log of four to five days' worth of eating in a diary, and I give them my analysis and tell them the truth about what the food they are consuming is doing or not doing to reach their goal. Their answer is always the same, "I don't eat as well as I thought." So here is a list of what are the most common things people think are healthy foods, but really aren't.

First, low fat dairy

There are numerous reasons why dairy isn't healthy, but to simplify — it is a highly-processed food that is both inflammatory and highly glycemic. This is due to the process of pasteurization and homogenization where milk is heated to sterilize it, then filtered to remove the fat globules. And because heat kills nutrients and damages the proteins and probiotics, it then needs to be fortified with synthetic man-made vitamins and minerals to replace the damage done during processing. Your body now recognizes this as an invader, not as a real nutrient dense food, thus causing inflammation and disruption in the digestive tract. By removing all the fat, there is nothing for the villi in the lining in the intestines to bind to that would slow the absorption into the blood stream and allow the body to break down the nutrients and utilize them, thus making it as highly glycemic as sugar and water. Not an ideal food to stabilize blood sugar. Opt for raw or organic full fat dairy, if you need to have it. It is a better and more satisfying choice.

Soy

Another highly marketed food that has people brainwashed into thinking it's a health food is soy. Not only is soy a neurotoxin, and most soy consumed is genetically modified, it is also a component that mimics estrogen. This causes hormonal disruption, but research also indicates that it causes early puberty when infants are given soy-based formulas. Women can experience menstrual irregularities while men can experience lower testosterone due to elevated estrogen production. Unless soy is organic and fermented it contains heavy levels of phytates. Phytates support nature by not allowing a seed, nut or grain to germinate until the environment has just the right amount of water and warmth to support life. The phytates do this by blocking enzyme (life) activity. Once the environment reaches the conditions for optimal survival, the phytates actively break down and the enzymatic processes trigger life to begin. Phytates are also mineral blockers and have been found to block absorption of zinc, calcium, selenium, iron and other minerals when consumed by humans. Even minor iron deficiencies can lead to fatigue, lethargy, poor athletic performance, a weakened immune system, and learning disabilities. These facts should be enough to convince you to avoid this stuff, but if you *Google* this info, you will find much more.

Gluten-free

Other products tainted by the food industry are gluten-free products. Yes, I am a big advocate of avoiding gluten whenever possible (even if you do not have celiac disease) because most products containing gluten have little or no nutritional value and are considered just empty calories in my book. Gluten (like phytates) also blocks the absorption of beneficial nutrients. Reason enough to avoid, with the price of good food what it is. So just like the fat-free craze of the 90s, big manufacturers are jumping on the bandwagon and flooding the market with gluten-free products. Even without the gluten these products are highly processed, and now contain extra sugars, fillers, binding agents, and a whole host of ingredients you can't pronounce. Mainly because of this, and also because gluten free products don't taste that great, my advice is to avoid all processed foods as much as possible, and just eat the real thing.

Drinks

The last item I want to shed light on is flavored and / or sports drinks. If you want to add quick pounds around your waist, start drinking your calories, or should I call it what it is — liquid chemicals. Think about what they give underweight patients and babies. Concentrated liquid calories. Look at heavy beer drinkers. Very few are thin because it is easy to drink mass amounts of calories in a short amount of time. Look at the label on sports drinks and juices and calculate the per serving calories you are consuming. Now realize that intense activity burns about 10 calories per minute. Now, do the math. Most are disguised as nutritional by inserting words such as "electrolyte, minerals, vitamins, 100 percent fruit, and protein," when in all actuality, you are drinking pasteurized, sugar added junk food. Unless you are juicing at home and you know all the ingredients, stay away from this stuff. If it says low or zero calories, it's even worse for you because it is all carbonated chemicals. And if its electrolytes you are looking for, just add a pinch of sea salt to your water. Electrolytes require minerals such as sodium, not sugar.

Keep a diary

You'll be surprised what foods you are eating, as well as what foods you are missing. Don't trust labels... read the back of the packages and avoid the front health claims. Learn more about what you put in your body and be skeptical about health claims. As with many things in life, there are few easy solutions.

15

LOSING SUMMER, NOT FITNESS

Here comes that time of year again. Summer is over, it's time to put the beach chairs away, cover the pool and grill, put away the patio furniture, hang the bikes in the garage, and swap out the skimpy tight clothing for heavier, looser-fitting, warmer stuff. It's the time of the year to bake apple pies, eat comfort food, and throw your hands in the air and blame the holidays and bad weather for your weight gain and physical demise. If this is you, I say you are making a big mistake.

It has been scientifically proven that light deprivation, due to shorter sunlight hours, causes depression and Vitamin D deficiency. And due to change, it is a biological defense mechanism to store more body fat so people in our region can keep warm. But with all that being said, good health and physical activity should not be seasonal, it should be a way of life. I realize that you need to turn up the intensity in the Spring because you want to peak and look your best for the Summer, and eating and training at a higher than normal level is not sustainable for most, but you should never completely stop. Pro athletes train differently when the season starts, off season, and pre-season, and so should we. In our "off" season, we still need to focus on our health and fitness even though there are a lot of distractions, and the desire diminishes.

Find your motivation

You need to find reasons to maintain what you work so hard for. One reason may be a winter getaway to somewhere warm, or if you ski or take part in other winter activities, or just the need for the strength and stamina to shovel snow, are all perfect examples of why you should stay in top physical condition. Here are a few things you can do to sustain. Join Providence Fit Body Boot Camp, or a Fit Body Boot Camp near you. Hire a personal trainer or coach to motivate you. When you pay for something, and put the appointment in the book, you are more likely to stick with the commitment. If you decide to do it on your own, I recommend joining a gym that offers programs that guarantee results and hold you accountable. Otherwise, you tend to get distracted at home or in an overwhelming facility. I would also recommend the local YMCA. I notice a few of them have been updated and they offer a lot of activities for the family. Another option would be to sign up at a small studio that offers yoga, Pilates, boxing for fitness, or various other activities. There is no reason to let your health suffer when there are fun options available.

16

LOSING WEIGHT
(GETTING FIT)
EASY AS 1-2-3?

#1 — Change Nutrition Habits
#2 — Start Moving
#3 — Progressions on numbers 1 & 2

Yes, these three steps are not glamorous, and not complicated, but they will take you to where you want to be — which is to be fitter and at an ideal weight. To lose weight (and get fit), you need to start with both mental and physical toughness. And… you need to set goals.

If you follow these three steps, you can expect to lose two to three pounds per week until you reach your ideal body weight. At that point, you will look and feel so much better. It becomes effortless, and you have not only reached that weight goal, but you have established new habits — habits that you have now adopted towards a healthy way of living. I don't believe in quick fixes — no pills, packaged food, liquid diets, point systems, etc. I do believe in motivation, in wanting "it" badly, and in having the discipline to change for the better. Saying that, let's start with the three steps.

Step #1 - Change your nutrition habits

For many of you who are overweight, this will mean an overhaul of your nutrition program. First, we start by changing the quality of your food. If you eat potato chips, substitute organic corn chips. If you eat a commercial yogurt, we swap for an organic / biodynamic farm yogurt with live cultures. We switch conventional vegetables and meats for organic. The reason we do this is because our bodies work more efficiently when we detox from elements such as cheap vegetable and canola oils, overly processed dairy, nitrates, corn syrup, soy, wheat, and other GMO fillers, as well as pesticides that cause major inflammation in the body. This step is by far more important than counting calories (which is the third progression after eliminating certain foods).

Step #2 — Get moving.

Try to move more whenever you can. Take the stairs if you are only going a few flights, park further away from the door, take a walk in your neighborhood or during lunch time at work. It is important to move to keep your system working properly, to help blood flow to extremities, release endorphins, stimulate digestion, release free radicals, and improve sleep as well as burn calories and feel more energetic. This is your body's jump start if you have been sedentary too long. You do not have to join a gym or do anything too strenuous at this point. This is to get the body acclimated to movement. If you do too much, you could become excessively sore or injured, and that will only discourage you and give little incentive to follow through on your program. That's why I believe in progressions. Start small, make attainable goals that you can reach, log your progress, and after a while it will become almost automatic.

Step #3 — Progressions on numbers 1 and 2

Focusing on exercise and nutrition are the only ways to lose weight and keep it off, but you will need to expand and make adjustments to your program when you reach plateaus. After a while, your body adapts to the changes you are making, so we need to make progressions. Here are some examples of progressions for your eating plan.

After you make the quality change, it's time to eliminate even more processed foods. Though they say they are organic and gluten-free, many of these foods are highly processed, and the less you eat of them the better. Make the transition to whole foods exclusively. The next thing to do when you reach a sticking point is calorie control. Everybody has different requirements and needs so you need to play with portion sizes. By this point you should have a good understanding of your body's needs, and how it reacts to dietary changes, so make some adjustments. Progression in exercise is endless. You can move from mild to intense by adding heavier loads and faster training. Go from walking to strength training to super setting to metabolic training to sprinting. This requires some common sense so do not overdo it. The best advice I can give on this one is to feel it out and listen to your body, train within your limits, but also push yourself. If still confused, hire a professional. Personal trainers can work with you on making your workout program adjust so your body doesn't acclimate to it, and some trainers have the expertise to also work with you on your nutrition changes. Losing weight and getting fit might not be "easy," but it is simply — 1, 2, and 3.

17

MAKING A LIST...
CHECKING IT TWICE!

How about a puppy? Or, a kitten? I know... a Lexus wrapped up with a big red bow? Nah... give the most valuable gift of all — give the gift that pays you back... the gift of fitness and health.

Let's face it, the holidays are a stressful time for most people. Why? Because most people are doing it all wrong. The holidays should be a time to relax and enjoy family, friends, and some good food and drink, not a time you should be getting pulled in different directions, fighting for parking spots at the mall, wondering what to buy people, and doing damage to your body by excessively drinking and eating. But a lot of us do it, and a lot of us later regret it when we are eight to twelve pounds heavier and need to make some stupid resolution that we will probably never keep.

Festive food

Not this year! Here are a few tips that will keep you sane, and fit through the holiday season. First of all, stick to your healthy nutrition plan. Keep up the meal frequency and you won't be hungry. You should be on a plan that has you eating "small and nutritious" snacks every three hours. We do this to keep our metabolism high, and to avoid extreme hunger. When you are hungry, you will more likely make a bad decision or overeat. Stay the course, and keep preparing your healthy holiday meals.

Party time

If you are going to a party or holiday dinner, eat something good first. Have a protein drink, piece of chicken, or some raw nuts. This will also help you limit the amount of damage you do when you arrive at your destination.

Drink and be merry

Alternate alcohol with water. Have a drink, but make round two a glass of water. "The solution for pollution is dilution." Drink lots of water when you drink booze, and you will consume less and feel better the next day. Hydrate those muscles that you worked so hard for.

Presents

When buying presents, think health. Here are a few ideas that some of your friends and family might appreciate:

Gift cards from stores like Whole Foods or other organic, natural retailers (do your research!) There's nothing better than getting to the register and not peeling off those bills or swiping that credit card.

Gift baskets. Make it more personal. Make up a gift basket with items such as olive oil, nice vinegar, and some unique spices. It's better than giving someone a basket of cookies and chocolates. Or even liquor. You think you are being generous, but you are not really helping someone with that type of gift.

Fitness gear. Another great gift for someone who already works out is fitness gear. The nicer stuff from Lululemon is pretty expensive, so some people won't spend that kind of money on themselves, but they make a nice gift. Stores like REI are also a great spot to find great gifts for your fitness enthusiast friends and family.

Memberships. If and only if someone wants to join a gym should you give them a gift of a membership. Working out and getting in shape is something you need to want to do, and giving someone a gift for a gym membership is not only a waste, but could be insulting. This is something they need to mention before you take action. If someone has mentioned that they want to belong to a gym, then cash towards a membership or a few personal training sessions is a great gift idea.

So be a little creative, and give a gift that will do some good for someone. Nice food baskets, gym gear, and maybe memberships will bring long lasting joy to someone's holiday, and keep them healthy all year. So, take out the shopping list again, give it another look, make some healthy changes — and be creative!

18

DON'T "SABOTAGE"
YOUR HOLIDAYS

I t's that time of the year again. A time to get together with family and friends who you don't get to see on a regular basis, a time to be close with the ones we love and care about, a time to give thanks, a time of relaxing and enjoying that warm feeling that the holidays bring.

But beware. The holidays don't always come with good intentions. As a matter of fact, the holidays love to "sabotage" our health and waistline. Here are some ways to avoid this.

> sab·o·tage, n
>
> 1. Destruction of property or obstruction of normal operations, as by civilians or enemy agents in time of war; 2. Treacherous action to defeat or hinder a cause or an endeavor; deliberate subversion.

S — stick to your exercise routine. Eating well is difficult this time of year, so don't compound the damage by being lazy. Get to the gym and lift weights.

A — avoid eating the worst of the food on the table. Stay away from all bread based foods like stuffing, bread, rolls, crackers etc. These items have the emptiest calories of all.

B — be strong. Don't eat just because it is in front of you. When you feel full, stop eating.

O — offer to help clean off the table and get up and move around after dinner. It is not a lot of exercise, but still better than sitting at the table spooning more food into your mouth.

T — take responsibility for yourself. If you look for reasons to give in and fail, you will. Don't just throw your hands in the air and blame your host or the holidays for falling off your program. We all cheat, just get back on the wagon after it's over.

A — accept the fact that you will *not* be on your program, and you *will* have dessert. This is for the neurotic exercise people. Don't stress yourself out, it's OK, just try to minimize the damage. You work hard, you deserve a treat.

G — get back to the gym tomorrow. Most people get this day off, so get to the gym the next day. You could also workout outside, but you will have lots of stored glycogen from overeating, and a workout with weights will burn more calories as well as give you a great pumped up feeling.

E — exercise discipline, and keep your motivation. When you fall off for a day get back on your horse. Try to avoid throwing in the towel for "the holiday season." There will be lots of temptation, but remember how hard you worked to get to where you are, and that the more you vary from your plan and system, the tougher it is to get back on track.

19

FIT FOR LIFE — YES, YOU!

Y column is titled, FIT FOR LIFE — and though I didn't come up with this name to describe my life, I really do live by that phrase. Health and fitness shouldn't be something that is seasonal, or done in cycles. It should be a way of life. The statistics in this country are alarming: approximately 65 percent of the population is overweight. This means that when you are in a crowd of people, you can see people who have a few extra pounds to lose. They may have a little flab around the midsection, or a little jiggle in their arms, or a little cellulite around their legs. So, basically if you are not in shape, you might be considered overweight. But over 33 percent of these people are obese. This is really very different. This means that you are carrying 35 percent or more of your body weight in fat pounds. And this figure is increasing every year. But it's also important to remember that these are just statistics that revolve around weight and muscle to fat ratios.

When I do a presentation, I always ask the crowd to raise their hands if they know someone who has had cancer or diabetes, and every time, about 99 percent of the crowd raises their hands. And although I like to be right most of the time, when these hands go up, for that moment, it stuns me. What is depressing and frustrating is that I believe this doesn't need to be. Science is showing us this doesn't need to be. Science is shouting at us that we are causing our own diseases, in large part, by behaviors that are controllable and modifiable.

The American Heart Association's slogan used to be "Your Life Is in Your Hands" and that just about said it all. There are hundreds of books about getting fit on the market. There are gyms around every corner, and then you have the internet. The information is out there, and people are spending billions of dollars a year trying to get fit and healthy. Sure, a lot of people don't care, and those who choose to ignore the facts are choosing to do harm to their bodies. For the most part, my focus has to be on the ones who want help, but can't figure out what to do to get to their optimal health. They're buying book after book, joining gyms, even hiring trainers, trying fad diets, and going to extremes to get in shape, but fitness still seems to elude them.

Why is this? Being fit is actually easy. I know I do it for a living, but that's why I consider it easy. Drink clean water, get eight hours of sleep, eat clean organic non-processed food, and move your body. That's it. You do not need complicated restrictive diets, you do not need to watch YouTube for complex and difficult exercises, and you do not need to read every diet book out there. All you need to do is follow my advice above.

OK! BUT... (I know what you are thinking, "Ha, I knew there was a catch.") The only way to achieve your goals is to do it CONSISTENTLY. Occasionally, eating right and moving around won't cut it. I hear it all the time, "I ate great for breakfast and lunch, but had a drink and a piece of cake, or some bread after work." This behavior is inconsistent, and will not net results. You need to eat well 90 percent of the time, and if you are consistent with a proper eating plan, then your ratio should look like this:

Eat 5 times a day (snacks and meals) for 7 days = 35 meals / snacks x 90 percent = just 3 1/2 bad meals, but 31 1/2 have to be healthy balanced meals to make progress.

In addition, you need to move around regularly. Even if you eat well, sitting all day leads to poor posture, and tight hips, usually causing lower back pain. You don't need to train like a marine every day, but you need to move consistently or you won't move efficiently.

Simplicity is the best way to go. Follow the few steps I have given you. Find a program that will work for you. Keep it simple, but follow it consistently. Just like building a house, the better you follow the plans, and the more time you put in on a regular basis, the faster it gets done. Building it is a smooth process, and maintenance makes it look great and it ensures it will last a long time.

20

ONE EXTRA DEGREE MAKES ALL THE DIFFERENCE.

At 212 degrees, water will boil. At 211, nothing happens. Above 212, water turns to steam that could power a locomotive. One degree is all it takes to make a difference.

This applies to your fitness and health routine as well. You can eat clean all day, consume five healthy meals, and then go home and eat a piece of bread, have a glass of wine, and just like that, your progress halts. That's it. It only takes one degree to determine the outcome of your progress, or lack thereof. On the other hand, if you exercised one more degree of effort every day, and didn't cheat at night, you can count on being a couple of pounds lighter on the scale at the end of the week, feel a little tighter, and see the shape of your abs a little better.

Everything in moderation is OK

I hear this all the time, but people have no concept what moderation is. Two glasses of wine at night isn't moderation. One glass a night isn't either. At 80 calories of sugar, times 7 nights, that's 560 extra calories a week. That's not moderation. If you happen to have a drink or two at a special occasion one or two times a month, you can call that moderation, but when you have a daily habit of eating

319

a piece of candy, or a piece of bread, it is not moderation — it is consistently screwing up a little bit at a time which will add up and derail your success.

Someone was coaxing one of my clients on social media into have Easter candy, saying, "just do it, you can work out harder and burn it off." This really upsets me because this guy kept justifying why he thought it was OK. Why would you eat a piece of garbage candy when you work so hard to make progress on the goals that are so important to you? Why put yourself in a position that will put you at a disadvantage? (By the way, this guy is out of shape, so misery loves company, I suppose.) It would be like driving recklessly to get somewhere and getting pulled over, getting a ticket, then driving twice as fast to get to your destination when you would have gotten there sooner if you just drove the speed limit. Instead, you stressed yourself out, lost money, and got an unfavorable result. It doesn't make any sense. Just exercise one more degree of discipline, and you will get a favorable result, with the same or less effort.

How you do anything is how you do everything

Think about that. Let it resonate. Then self-assess. You will find this statement true. Maybe not to your liking, but it is true. If you fail at something like your nutrition, you justify it by saying, "a little won't hurt me." Do you see yourself justifying or having an excuse for everything you know you are doing wrong? If you habitually hit the snooze button in the morning, you probably are not prepared for the day. You most likely are late much of the time, playing catch up, or are stressing and rushing to be on time. If your house is a mess, your car and desk probably are too. So is your pocketbook and briefcase? If you lack structure and discipline in your life, you are probably find yourself not in good physical condition either, because your nutrition and exercise routine require both of these.

If you are a negative person, you probably complain about everything from politics to the person waiting on your table. You lay the blame on everyone else when things don't work out in your favor at work, at home, and everywhere you go. If someone earns more than you, it's the boss playing favorites, not your bad work ethic.

However, if you are disciplined, and have structure in your life, you are probably a go-getter and over-achiever. You are probably in good physical shape, you earn more than your co-workers, and you get important things done. You have an easier time putting your mind to something, making a plan, and accomplishing your goals at the end of the day.

It's all about mindset

Whether you are in a good position health-wise, financially, mentally, spiritually, or you know you're not — the good news is that you can make a change. It's all what you put your mind to. Remember your actions are controlled by thought, and your body does what your mind tells it to do. So, the next time you feel frustrated that you are not where you want to be, don't give up. You are worth the effort! If others can achieve, you can too. Set your mind right, and remember, one more degree of effort in whatever it is you are doing will result in a positive change. Program yourself, set goals, think positive, and go that extra degree.

21

SIZE MATTERS

If a little bit is good, why is too much better? News flash... it's not. But we, as Americans, seem to think so. Look around and read the signs. *Supersize, Big Gulp, Extreme, Huge, Extra, Insanity, Giant Size, 20 Percent Larger e* — you see these descriptions on everything from food and drinks to exercise products. So why are manufacturers using these descriptions to sell products? Because we, as Americans, have become spoiled and lazy. When you over indulge in something you become a glutton, and tend to overdo everything. We are spoiled because everything is easily accessible, and easy to get. This is why we are in the state we are in with all the disease, obesity, and position in the world. We feel entitled to have more.

Why we do what we do

Why pay $10 for a quality meal, when you can get twice as much cheap garbage-food for the same price? Is it value we are after, or do we feel we deserve bigger for the same money? Isn't a regular size cup of soda enough? Nah, let's get a Big Gulp, because you get more. Eight ounces of meat is enough to eat at one sitting. Yet when you look at a menu, there is always the 22-ounce option for a few dollars more. And there are those who will order it. Why? Eight ounces carries over 50 grams of protein, more than enough for the biggest bodybuilder to metabolize at one time, but people still go for the "bigger" option. It's not because we are all that hungry, because I guarantee if everyone cut back to normal portion sizes and ate or consumed only what the body needed, they would still be satisfied. It's the "more" attitude we have adopted. You could blame the food industry, but they are doing their job — capitalizing on demand, and making huge money at any expense, even if it means having a negative effect on much of the nation, especially our kids. Drug dealers and Big Pharma, it can be said, are on much of the same level. They have no soul, scruples, or care about the damage left behind. Because the only thing that matters is the money. And Americans are falling victim to it all. On the other hand, nobody is tying people down and forcing them to consume these products. We do have choice. We can control our size portions and the food and drink we consume. So, should we just consume and lay blame? Or, take accountability for ourselves and our family? Be strong and do the right thing. And don't blame ignorance because the information is out there.

Do just enough.

There are over 40 COUNTRIES, yes, countries, not states, that ban GMO foods. Yet only 24 states in THIS country have eliminated the use of these products. Why is this? It is all about the money, and we are gobbling it up. Pun intended. But let's be fair about this whole overindulgence thing. It's not just the overweight and obese, the fitness people are guilty, too. If a little exercise is good, then more must be better so some people think. I look at exercise like food, if you don't eat enough, your body will not respond to new muscle growth, or perform at its peak potential. If you eat too much, you gain too much body fat, but when you dial in your nutrition plan, the results will ALWAYS be favorable. The same goes for exercise. Not enough, and the results will not be there, but if you exercise too much, or at too high a rate of an intensity, the results are disastrous.

My philosophy is exercise just enough to achieve your goal. No more, no less. An example of this mindset would be if you are training for an Ironman competition, you need to take it to the extremes, but if you are just trying to get in better shape, and lose a few pounds, you do not need to beat your body sore for days. I see it all the time — regular working people, just trying to get fit, abusing their bodies to the point of injury. I allow my members unlimited access to the sessions on my schedule, yet when I see someone taking too many in a row, I try to explain the pitfalls of over training, such as muscle breakdown, hormonal imbalance, adrenal fatigue, and finally injury. I also ask the question, "how well can you perform in everyday life if you are injured? Not well, or not at all?"

So, let's use some common sense when choosing an exercising program, and pick one that pushes you out of your comfort zone but not beyond your ability. Make sure you are mildly sore in the right places, and are able to perform your everyday life tasks. Train hard but train smart. If the program you choose has the words extreme, insanity, or killer in the title, make sure you are capable of handling the outcome.

22

THERE'S GOT TO BE A MORNING AFTER

O K, so yesterday happened. You had a great time with family, friends and assorted loved ones and much joy was had by all. It was a beautiful day.

Aaannndddd… you ate like crap.

If you are like most of my clients (and yes, like me, too) you ate too much, you ate "bad" things, and probably drank more than normal, too. Now, you wake up this morning looking a bit more like Santa than you did just a day ago. Thank you — food hangover!

Damage control

So now what? It's time to go into damage control mode. But here's the good news: It's way easier than you think. Take a breath and follow these simple tips to get back on track without going crazy.

1. Don't beat yourself up

You need to keep this in mind. One bad meal (or one bad day of eating) will not make you fat just like one good day of eating will not make you lean. It is what we do long term that makes the difference. So pick yourself up, dust yourself off, and move forward.

2. Don't weigh yourself

Don't go near a scale. At least not today. A couple of things happen when you pig out. One is you just retain water from the increased overall consumption and salt intake. And another is you fill up your glycogen stores (the sugar stored in muscle). Now that in and of itself is just fine, but with every gram of glycogen stored, two to three grams of water is stored. Again, that is not bad thing but that will increase the number on the scale. So avoid the freak-out and avoid the scale.

3. Stick with P & P

"P&P" is just an easy way to remember protein and produce. To put it simply, carbs can problematic for a lot of people. They can make you gain fat and can keep you from losing fat (this has to do with their influence on insulin). So, to get your nutrition in check, stick with protein and produce. The protein helps increase metabolism and helps muscle repair. Fresh vegetables can give your body all the nutrients it needs plus has a ton of fiber to keep you full. There are some other important nutritional aspects to consider, but if you get these two things rolling, you are moving in the right direction.

4. Hydrate

Here's a secret. Increased water intake does not increase fat loss. *BUT* even the slightest bit of dehydration stops fat loss in its tracks. And add to that the fact your body only functions optimally when it is fully properly hydrated. Aim for around a gallon per day. And yes, you'll be in the bathroom a lot.

5. Get moving

Get off your butt. Now. Anything is better than nothing, even just going for a walk. But if you want to get the most efficient fat torching workouts stick with short duration interval based training. In only 30 minutes, you can boost your metabolism for over 48 hours, melting fat even while at rest.

6. You can't fix it all today

Remember, you can't fix all your problems in a day, or even in a week. Dedicate yourself to yourself. This is the only body you have, and your future self will thank you for the time and effort you invest in yourself now. It will not happen overnight, but it will happen when you commit to change your life. It is never too late, and trust me: You are worth it.

See, it's really not that tough. Also, I am here for you. So, if you need any help and guidance, if you have questions or need some someone to amp up your motivation, just get in touch and I'll help you out. Now — get ready — New Year's Eve is right around the corner!

23

WEALTHY? HEALTHY? OR BOTH!

I am always hearing about how being healthy costs more than being unhealthy, and that you have to be wealthy to be healthy. Well, there is some truth to this, because everything in life in general is easier with a large bankroll. But I am going to give you some tips on how to overcome the expense and explain the pay off.

Most of the people that complain the loudest are the ones shopping at big box stores and looking for deals on food. When I occasionally visit this type of store, I observe what is in shoppers' baskets and carriages and I always see cases of juice and junk food purchased in bulk. This is the type of wasteful spending that is going to impact the cost of shopping in a negative way. Some good news here is that these stores are jumping on the organic and health food band-wagon, so you can still get some better prices on food than the smaller stores, but you will probably end up buying a bunch of stuff you don't need. I use these big discount stores for non-perishable items such as paper goods. I recommend shopping for your food on a weekly basis and purchasing fresh stuff.

Don't (always) listen to your mother

My mother is notorious for buying larger quantities of meat and freezing what she doesn't immediately need. I find fault with this for two reasons. First, frozen food doesn't taste as good, and second, I watch as she regularly throws stuff away. You forget it's there and it gets freezer burn or gets old. Imagine a stocked freezer and losing power in your house — there goes hundreds of dollars down the drain. When you pay a little more for food and you buy only what you need, it all averages out. Buying in bulk is not necessary. You do not need to store food. We are in no danger of a shortage! Buy fresh and shop frequently.

Like money in the bank!

When you look at the big picture, shopping healthy actually pays off — in big ways. First, you spend less when you shop. Rather than buying cases, you only buy what you need. Now look at the long-term savings: most OTC drugs won't be needed because when you eat correctly you breathe better, so allergy meds are needed far less often. Your joints ache less, so you probably won't need the anti-inflammatory stuff. Your sex drive is still there so you don't need to buy ED drugs! Your headaches and other symptoms that eating wholesome, good food prevents will become non-existent, you will be more productive and ambitious, and that pays off in your ability to work better and make more money. So, the next time you are in the checkout line at the organic quality market, remember you are not overpaying for food, you are making an investment — in yourself. And that's as good as money in the bank.

24

THE FOOD WE EAT

Recently, I asked my followers on Facebook to tell me what topics they were interested in reading about, learning more about, and hearing my opinions and advice about. More than fitness, I heard there were lots of questions about whole foods, natural foods, what organic means, what GMOs are, what I should eat, and where I should shop. There is so much confusion today. Are labels accurate? What's the difference between what you read on the front of packaging and what is on the label — and how do you read a label?

You can't exercise out a bad diet

When people begin to work with me to attain better fitness, one of the first things I offer to do is to take them shopping. We learn about "whole" foods and eating organic, or as near to organic as possible. We talk about going "back to basics" and natural foods prepared in natural, wholesome ways. Watch how you prepare your foods and eat as natural as you can. You might even start by growing your own foods, then taking what's growing now in your gardens and bringing them inside for the cold season. There's no reason you can't continue to have fresh herbs and other items all year round.

The GMO issue & labeling

What are GMOs? A genetically modified organism (GMO) is an organism whose genetic material has been altered using genetic engineering techniques. Organisms that have been genetically modified include micro-organisms such as bacteria and yeast, insects, plants, fish, and mammals. GMOs are the source of genetically modified foods, and are also widely used in scientific research and to produce goods other than food. Genetic modification involves the mutation, insertion, or deletion of genes. Over 60 countries have banned or restricted the production or sale of GMOs. They include Australia, Japan, and all of the European nations, but so far, no ban exists in the U.S.

As far as labeling goes, while products currently do not have to disclose if they contain GMO ingredients, they can note that they don't — you'll see the label usually on the front of the product: "Non-GMO." This is similar with RBGH found in dairy. You'll see some cartons marked "No RBGH." Locally, both Maine and Connecticut have passed laws requiring GMO labeling. Some food companies, such as Whole Foods, have partnered with the "Non-GMO Project" to independently verify which food items are non-GMO, with full labeling targeted for 2017.

Why GMOs?

Originally, GMOs were used as a way to keep growing foods healthier; as an herbicide. They were used to produce GMO corn, soy, and other basic food crops. No one knows the long-term impact of GMOs in our food chain. There is much we do not know, but much to concern us, so I still go with some basic advice. If you want to be sure there are no GMOs in your food pantry, buy "organic." Look for "No GMOs" on your food labels. Watch what you add to your foods to prepare them — oils, in particular. Think about that home garden. Read more about the issue. I've listed some good sources for more information, below. I like this advice the best, "if the food would not have been found in my grandma's kitchen, then it won't be found in mine."

I want to thank you for reading this book and I hope it helps you unleash your full potential.

I am a firm believer that everybody has the opportunity to succeed in whatever their mission is, but it takes the right mindset, discipline and work ethic for it to become a reality.

My best advice is to never stop trying to develop and self-improve. Always have the mindset that you will never peak and the best is yet to come. Follow this plan and there are no limitations to what you can accomplish.

Committed to your success,

"Coach" Matt

ABOUT THE AUTHOR

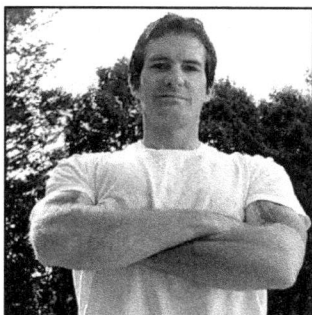

Matt Espeut is a resident of Providence, Rhode Island, and has been a personal trainer and nutrition consultant for over 25 years. He is the founder of **Fitness Profiles**, a one-on-one personal training company, and is the owner of **Providence Fit Body Boot Camp** located in Providence.

Matt influences the lives of others positively through his 5000 square-foot fitness and training facility, and by volunteering his time with different organizations like the Cub Scouts and the Shea High School football team in Pawtucket, Rhode Island where he has just completed his fourth year, helping the team to an undefeated season and state championship title. He is also paid coach with the city of Pawtucket, R.I.

Matt financially supports many different charities including Operation Stand Down, the American Cancer Society, The Autism Project, Teen Challenge, Nathan's Angels, and others. He also belongs to a charitable organization called Sweat Angels which matches his donations for every person who checks into his facility. The funds are donated to different charities such as Soles for Souls, Bricks for Schools, and other national efforts that Matt supports.

He also speaks to elementary and junior high school students as part of the annual "All-State Read" program created by author Joy Feldman.

In addition to training, volunteering, coaching, and writing, Matt does some free-lance modeling with Donahue Models and the Model Club of Boston. He also maintains active motivational and informative speaking programs.

www.ingramcontent.com/pod-product-compliance
Lightning Source LLC
Chambersburg PA
CBHW062156270326
41930CB00009B/1553